"Let food be thy medicine, a[nd medicine be thy food.]"

-HIPPOCR[ATES]

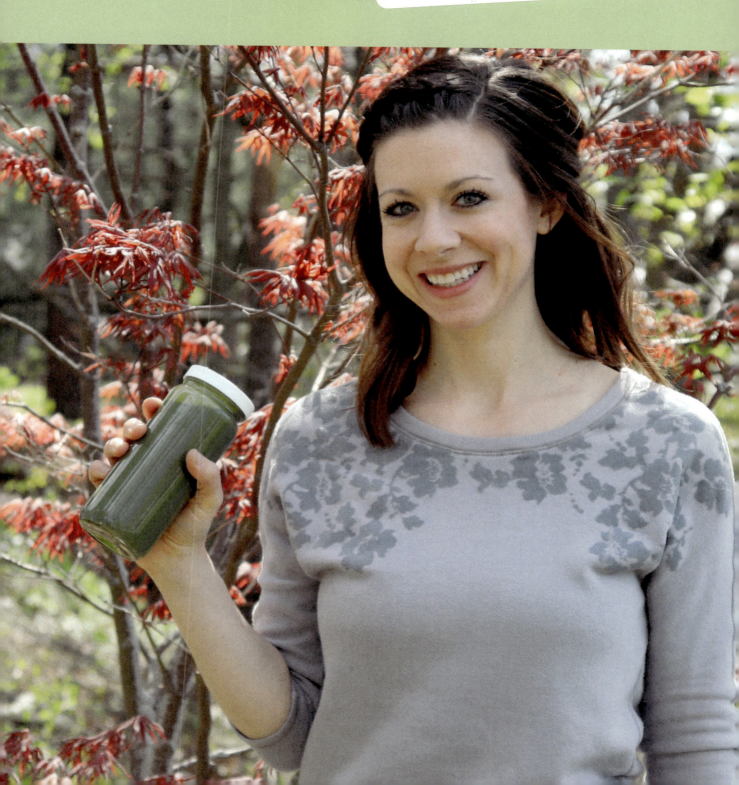

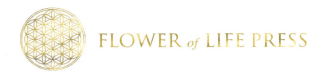

Plant-Based Vegan & Gluten-free Cooking with Essential Oils:
Your Kitchen Companion For A High-Vibe Life

Copyright © 2020 Lauren D'Agostino

All rights reserved. No part of this publication may be reproduced, distributed, or transmitted in any form or by any means, including photocopying, recording, or other electronic or mechanical methods, without the prior written permission of the publisher, except in the case of brief quotations embodied in critical reviews and certain other noncommercial uses permitted by copyright law.

Disclaimer: The advice herein is not intended to replace the services of trained health professionals or be a substitute for medical advice. You are advised to consult with your health-care professional with regard to matters relating to your health, and in particular matters that may require diagnosis or medical attention.

*These statements have not been evaluated by the Food and Drug Administration. The content in this book is not intended to diagnose, treat, cure, or prevent any disease.

Book design by **Astara Jane Ashley, flowerofflifepress.com**

Food Photos by **Katarina Gallagher @kngfood**

To contact the publisher, visit flowerofflifepress.com

Library of Congress Control Number: Available upon request

ISBN-13: 978-1-7337409-8-2

Printed in the United States of America

PLANT-BASED VEGAN & GLUTEN-FREE
COOKING WITH *Essential Oils*

YOUR KITCHEN COMPANION FOR A HIGH-VIBE LIFE

*Enjoy!
♡ Lauren*

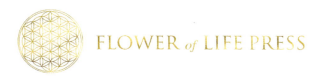

Praise

I love using essential oils in the more traditional ways and honestly felt intimidated to use them in my cooking...until now. Lauren has created simple and delicious recipes that make it so easy to use these beautiful oils in my cooking. No second-guessing myself anymore! And...you don't have to be vegan to love these recipes. I am not vegan but try to include as many plant-based foods as I can in our meals. The recipes in this book will become staples in our kitchen going forward. One of my favorite things about this cookbook is just how well organized and beautiful it is! I am so excited about this cookbook!

—Mary Shackelford, RN, HN-BC,
Holistic Wellness Practitioner

An all-natural approach to healing from the inside out, this book is such a great source of both information and inspiration. You don't have to be 100% committed to veganism to appreciate the value this cookbook has to offer. After spending time with Lauren, taking the photos for this book and taste testing these recipes, the skeptical veil was lifted off my eyes and I am now a believer in natural remedies.

—Katarina Gallagher, Pastry Chef and
Food Photographer @kngfood

Chef Lauren's take on plant-based cooking with essential oils is as inventive as it is practical. This cookbook invites you alongside her on a journey for culinary fulfillment. Inspiring for newbies and seasoned curmudgeons alike!

—Chef Scott Rawdon

This cookbook is filled with creative ways to flavor nutrition-packed food in an exciting and crowd-pleasing way! As a registered dietitian nutritionist, I work with many individuals who find it challenging to include plant-based foods. Chef Lauren's recipes are sure to inspire even the most skeptical eaters!

—Gina Rancourt, MS, RD, CD

Lauren is such a delight! I have had the pleasure of tasting some of her recipes and am blown away! She is very mindful in her approach, as she brilliantly repurposes as much of the plant and other ingredients in each recipe to ensure nothing goes to waste! She is extremely knowledgeable and passionate about using essential oils in the kitchen.

—Alisha Hanoian, Essential Oil Educator

What a gift! Lauren has combined her culinary talents with her knowledge as a Health Coach and essential oil expert to bring us something special! I've been using essential oils since 2012 and have always wanted to do more than put a drop in my water, hummus or on apple slices. Thank you, Lauren, for this treasure!

—Eileen Ladwig MS, OTR/L, Essential Oil Educator

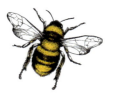

Lauren brings such a beautiful simplicity to an often overly complicated lifestyle. Her intentional approach to mindful, plant-based living is infused into each recipe. 'Plant-Based Vegan Cooking with Essential Oils' is a stunning testament to Lauren's dedication to holistic living, intuitive cooking and finding ritual and gratitude in the kitchen.

—Hannah Smith, LMT, INHC, YMT

This book really is the first of its kind. With the world becoming more aware of the benefits of plant-based diets, and the power of plants in general, this book should really be on every plant-based chef's countertop. Lauren has such a lovely way of making cooking and baking fun and easy, and these recipes just make me want to put down whatever I'm doing and head to the kitchen! Thank you for sharing your passion and knowledge with us and I look forward to trying every recipe.

—Mystie Ziminsky, Owner/Founder of Plantz Café, Dracut MA

I am very much intrigued by using essential oils to cook with as a means of healing the body. I'm a big fan of alternative medicine and when you can incorporate that idea into food as well, I'm all for it! I too am a private chef and I'm excited to try out some of Lauren's amazing recipes!

—Patricia B, Private Healthy Chef

Lauren is a gorgeous spirit and a plant-based chef goddess! Her ability to infuse her love for everything "high vibe", mixing it with plants and the highest quality essential oils and manifesting for us all to share is nothing short of inspirational. These essential oil-infused recipes surpass any I have seen collected before! I'm ecstatic she had the foresight and skill to ground her food miracles so we could all partake in the magic that is *Plant-based Vegan and Gluten-Free Cooking with Essential Oils*! I thank the luckiest of stars my retreat (and life) chef is found!

—Michelle Blanchette, Life, Yoga, and Breath Coach

Chef Lauren has managed to channel her fun passionate nature into this essential cookbook. For those looking to make a change to a healthier lifestyle who have felt intimidated about where to start this book makes it super easy and relatable! I love how the different sections are broken down so that you can reference why on an emotional or physical level each oil would be recommended for a recipe and how to achieve the flavor safely. These days it is hard to find recipes that someone with any level of cooking expertise could execute this book is now my go-to reference for all things plant-based!

—Tricia Utley, Owner of Tricia Utley Energy Esthetics

Dedication

To Mama Gaia.

Thank you for blessing this planet with your beautiful gifts.

Contents

Introduction 1
Chef Lauren's Story 9
About the Author 13

Part 1: Cooking with Herbal Oils 15

Basil 19
Cilantro 23
Lemongrass 27
Marjoram 33
Oregano 37
Rosemary 45
Thyme 49

Part 2: Cooking with Spice Oils 53

Black pepper 57
Cardamom 61
Cassia 65
Celery seed 69
Cinnamon bark 73
Clove 77
Coriander 81
Fennel 87
Ginger 91
Turmeric 95

Part 3: Cooking with Mint Oils 99

Peppermint 103
Spearmint 107

Part 4: Cooking with Citrus Oils 109

Bergamot 113
Grapefruit 117
Lemon 121
Lime 129
Tangerine 135
Orange 139

Part 5: Cooking with Floral Oils 145

Geranium 149
Lavender 151

Acknowledgments 154

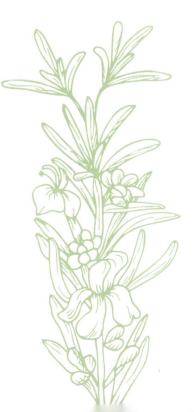

Contents by Recipe

Drinks + Smoothies

Blueberry basil lemonade 21
Masala chai 62
Bright green juice 87
Fresh ginger beer 93
Sore throat soother tea 93
Super juice 70
Peppermint hot cacao 103
Green detox smoothie 124
Raspberry lime rickey 131
Limeade with local honey 135
Blueberry muffin smoothie 140
Vanilla lavender moon milk 152
Lavender lemonade 153

Dressings + Marinades + Seasonings

Greens pesto 19
Cilantro lime dressing 23
Greek dressing 39
Oregano pesto 40
BBQ dressing 38
Almond ginger dressing 91
Fruit salad dressing 118
Lemon herb vinaigrette 124
Mexican seasoning salt 23
Green curry paste 28
Herbal marinade 37
Chimichurri 40
Rosemary balsamic marinade 45
Simple seasoning salt 57
Spicy coriander seasoning 84
Moroccan seasoning salt 83
Thai seasoning salt 25
Turmeric dressing 95
Citrus seasoning salt 130

Hummus + Veggies

Roasted tomato + carmelized onion spread 20
Fresh guacamole 24
Pico de gallo 23
Black bean lime hummus 129
Thai hummus 27
Spinach artichoke hummus 33
Quick pickles 71
Rainbow slaw 69
Lemon herb carrots 35
Italian marinated eggplant 49
Moroccan carrot hummus 77
Cauliflower with garlic, herbs, and vegan parmesan 84
Spiced roasted potatoes 83
Lemon garlic hummus 125
Mango lime salsa 129

Meat Substitutions + Mains

Vegan lentil meatballs 20
Coconut green curry braised jackfruit 28
BBQ braised jackfruit 38
Carnitas braised jackfruit 25
Herbed pasta 34
Spinach artichoke pasta 34
Pasta primavera 42
Marinated cauliflower steak 57
Lentil tikka masala 63
Lemony pasta with spinach + olives 122

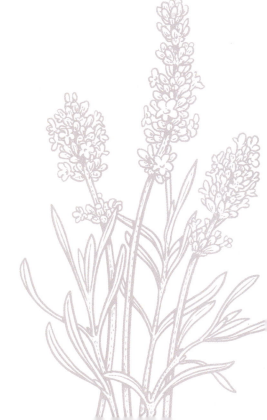

Contents by Recipe

Salads + Soups + Sauces

Apple, radish and plum salad..61
Celery and apple salad with walnuts 87
Celery salad with vinaigrette 70
Mojito berry watermelon salad...107
Kale salad with grapefruit 117
Roasted beet salad...118
Quinoa tabbouleh with lemon herb vinaigrette 125
Carrot salad with lime and cilantro 129
Thai butternut soup 31
Coconut red lentil curry..96
Squash + apple soup 81
Vegan clam chowder.. 51
Miso bowls...93
Express pasta sauce 37
Mushroom gravy...46
Sweet + sour stir fry 139

Sweets

Holiday glazed gingerbread 73
Sweet potato waffles... 74
Spiced coconut cream 75
Sweet potato pie..79
Chai frosted sweet potato cupcakes..78
Christmas cookie oat bites... 88
Peppermint cacao mousse 104
Mint chocolate chia pudding pops...103
Chocolate glazed peppermint bread 105
Chocolate peppermint cheesecake...105
Mint cacao chip nice cream 107
Earl grey tea cake.. 113
Citrus burst cheesecake 119
Lemon chia bread.. 121
Lemon burst cupcakes 126

Coconut lime cheesecake *130*
Creamsicle nice cream *135*
Cranberry orange bread *141*
Flower power pound cake *149*
Blueberry lavender bread *151*
Lavender chocolate truffles *152*
Cinnamon chocolate truffles *66*
Orange chocolate truffles *140*

Snacks

Pizza popcorn *41*
Rosemary popcorn *47*
Rosemary roasted walnuts *45*
Thyme roasted walnuts *51*
Black pepper roasted cashews *58*
Cassia roasted pecans *65*
Pumpkin spice popcorn *65*
Apple pie spiced popcorn *77*
Golden milk popcorn *95*
Roasted wasabi peanuts *91*
Tangerine roasted pistachios *135*
Honey orange roasted almonds *139*

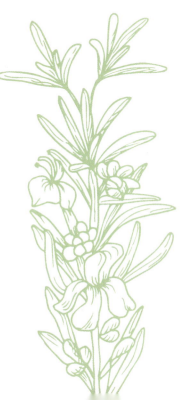

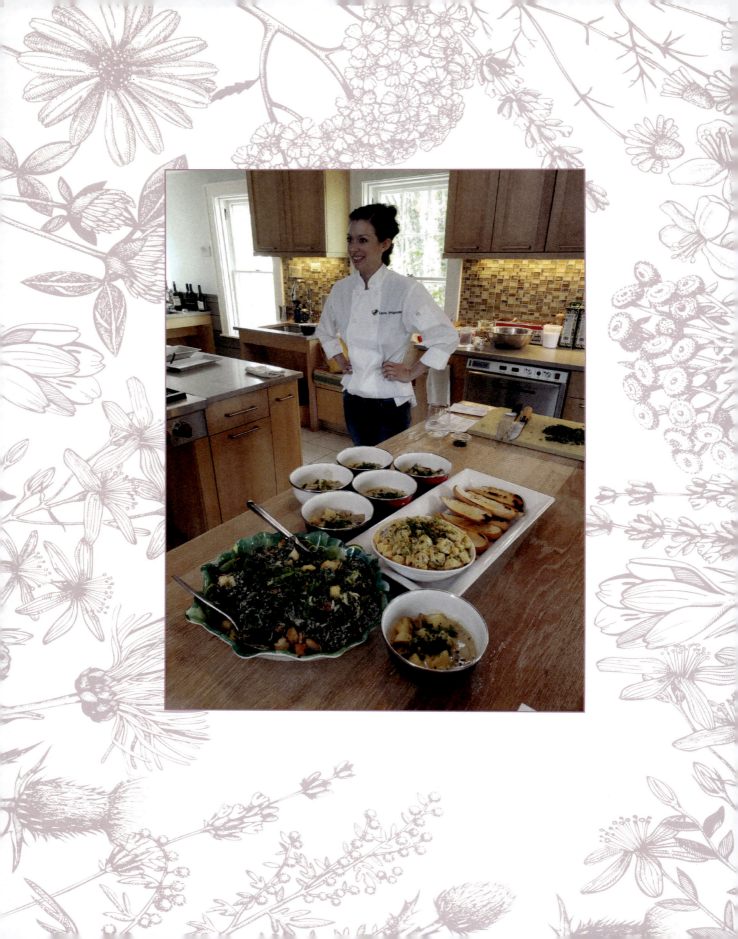

Introduction

It has been so much fun crafting the recipes in this book because I've truly come to appreciate the magic of these plants and their essential oils.

One of the most wonderful benefits of using certified pure therapeutic grade essential oils is their many uses, including internal consumption for those generally regarded as safe, or GRAS. Because plant-based eating and food preparation are such natural and integral parts of our lives, it's no surprise that essential oils extracted from the plants we commonly cook with can be used in the kitchen.

Before we dive into the exciting world of plant-based cooking with essential oils, let me preface these recipes with my personal culinary philosophy and how I became a different kind of chef, and then we'll make sure we're all on the same page with what essential oils are and how we use them in our homes, and most importantly, our kitchens.

Thank you...

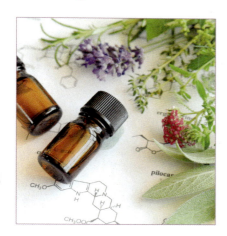

Discovering natural solutions with essential oils is so empowering and inspiring! Having these plant-based remedies right at your fingertips gives great peace of mind. Thank you for your openness to learning about this alternative form of healthcare, and cheers to your journey with natural remedies.

When I learned that I could also cook with these powerful oils, I was so intrigued by the flavors and experiences that I could create, with just one drop of oil! Thank you for your interest in learning to cook with essential oils.

Learning to cook from a young age is one of the best blessings in my life, and I believe it is something that every single person should know how to do for themselves. Feeding ourselves with meals that have been prepared purposefully, mindfully, and with high vibrations of love and gratitude is one of the most powerful forms of self-love I can think of. And what better gift than to be able to do this for yourself, and share this with loved ones?

And most importantly, thank you, thank you, thank you for having the courage to explore a new way of eating and caring for your body. Changing lifestyle habits is scary and hard, but here you are, and I thank you for joining me!

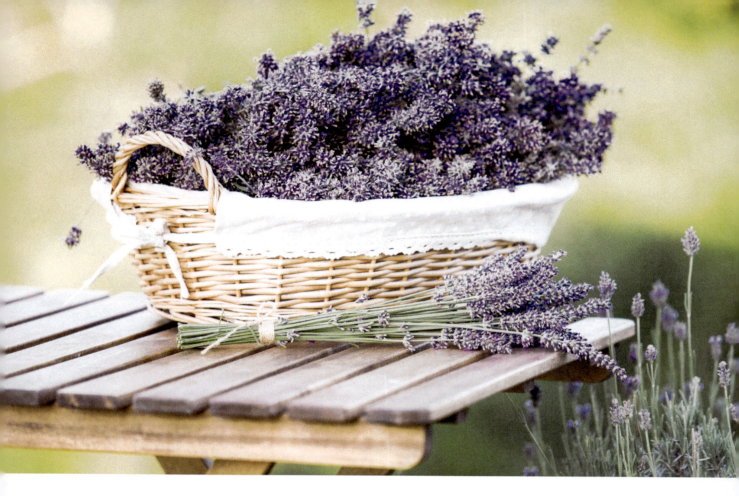

What are essential oils?

Essential oils are the natural aromatic compounds found in plants, flowers, herbs, bark, roots, and leaves. They give plants their distinct smell, help the plant heal, and repel pests or attract pollinators. Humans have been using these oils for thousands of years in their beauty rituals, for courage in times of war, and in spiritual healing practices. Nature has provided us with everything we need, and by harnessing the power of these essential oils, we are able to support our health and vitality in the many ways that nature intended.

It is important to note that not all oils are created equally. Many companies use synthetic ingredients, fillers, or other substances to extend the shelf-life or dilute their oils. It is so important to use oils that are pure, potent, and effective for the best results—it's a difference you can smell!

Before you use essential oils in your cooking, it is important to know how they have been produced, harvested, and distilled, and if they've been tested by the producer for possible contaminants or harmful substances. Because of the rise in popularity of essential oils, not all companies are committed to making sure that you are getting the most effective, most potent, and most pure essential oils.

Trusting that your oils are pure...

Not all essential oils are created equal, so to ensure that the oils you receive are always of the highest quality, it is important to know about the particular company's dedication to sourcing 100% pure, unadulterated essential oils. If they are strictly tested using third party labs, you can feel confident that you are using the very best oils for the health of you and your family.

Top brands will not sell anything that does not meet their highest standards so you can rest assured that each and every bottle you reach for will perform consistently and to the extent that is intended. Only the top essential oil brands use these testing processes to ensure that their essential oils are safe to use. During several rounds of rigorous testing, essential oils are closely examined to ensure that they don't contain any contaminants or harmful substances.

Pure oils are taken directly from natural sources and are harvested in optimal conditions by growers who are masters of their craft. These farmers have passed down their trade from generation to generation and their distilled oils do not contain processed or harmful ingredients. In fact, the oils are often distilled right in the community where the plant grows so that the farmers may receive fair and on-time wages.

Because essential oils are not regulated by the FDA, some companies add fillers and synthetic ingredients to their oils. When our bodies meet these synthetic oils, the desired effect of the oil may not be achieved and can sometimes do more harm than good. By choosing certified pure oils in your home and in your kitchen, you can enjoy the benefits, and peace of mind, of 100% natural essential oils.

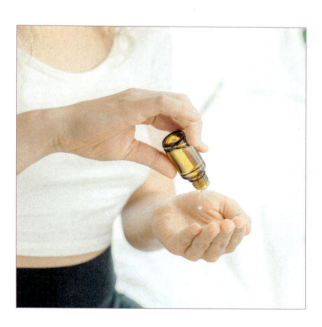
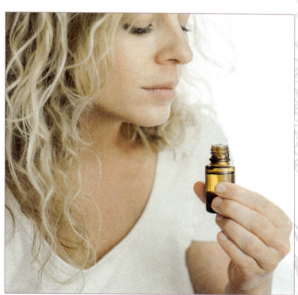

Generally recognized as safe

The FDA has compiled a list of substances that have been identified as "Generally Recognized as Safe," or GRAS, for use in food products. This list identifies substances that have substantial documentation of safe internal usage and includes essential oils.

The following oils are considered safe: basil, bergamot, black pepper, cassia, cinnamon, clary sage, fennel, geranium, ginger, grapefruit, juniper berry, lavender, lemon, lemongrass, lime, marjoram, melissa, oregano, peppermint, pink pepper, roman chamomile, rosemary, spearmint, tangerine, thyme, turmeric, orange, and ylang ylang.

Due to their chemical makeup, some essential oils should never be added to food or used internally. These oils and blends will not have the "Supplement Facts" panel on the bottle so no need to memorize! *The following oils are not safe for cooking:* arborvitae, cedarwood, cypress, douglas fir, eucalyptus, spikenard, white fir, and wintergreen.

Is it safe to consume essential oils?

Internal usage of essential oils has actually been practiced for centuries, and this is not a new concept or trend. The key to safe use is following proper safety guidelines, and always looking for the "Supplement Facts" panel on the side of the bottle. Like anything, essential oils only present risks when used improperly or in incorrect amounts.

Fruits, plants, and plant parts are already a natural and essential part of our diets, which makes it safe for our bodies to consume the oils since we are already well equipped to process them effectively. Like anything we consume, essential oils are ingested through the digestive system, enter the bloodstream, and are metabolized by the organs. Because our bodies recognize the essential oils as natural parts of our ideal human diet, they are easily processed and metabolized. Cooking with essential oils is simply a fun and convenient way to enrich the food we eat every single day.

How else do we use essential oils?

Essential oils can be enjoyed in three ways: aromatically, topically, and internally. Aromatic use is the most commonly thought of method, but it can be very beneficial to learn how to use these powerful oils safely both topically and internally.

Aromatic use means smelling and inhaling the essential oil through our sense of smell. This can be done by using a diffuser, or by simply dropping an oil into the palms and rubbing together before cupping around the nose and taking a few long, slow inhales.

Using essential oils topically means applying to the skin directly. Dilution is recommended for use with children, the elderly, and people with sensitive skin. Dilution does not diminish the effects of the essential oil; it simply distributes the essential oil over a larger surface area and increases absorption.

Use any carrier oil you like, such as fractionated coconut, jojoba, or avocado oil. This method can be effective when targeting a specific area such as sore knees, feet, back, or for absorption into a troubled area such as the abdomen for digestive support. Some oils have benefits related to the chakra areas as well, in which case applying to the intended area is useful. Applying oil to the bottoms of your feet, back of the neck, behind the ears, and insides of the wrists are great places for absorption into the body and through the sense of smell.

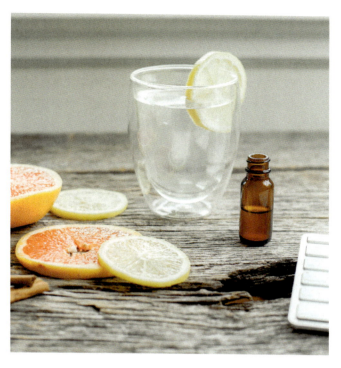

For internal use, it is important to use caution. Only oils with the supplement facts panel on the bottle are safe for internal consumption. Some oils like frankincense and peppermint can be dropped under the tongue. Other oils can be added to water for a pleasant experience, such as lemon or grapefruit. Oils that are commonly taken internally, such as Restful blend and Digestive blend are available in a convenient softgel form. Alternatively, you can easily make your own blend by using empty veggie caps and adding the oils of your choice.

You've likely been enjoying some internal benefits of essential oils without realizing it! The stomach calming effect of ginger, breath freshening power of peppermint, and lively flavor of fresh herbs are just some of the ways you have likely already enjoyed essential oils.

Why cook with them?

You might be wondering why you would want to cook with essential oils in the first place. Can't you just use the dried, ground, or fresh version of these plants and plant parts? The short answer is yes, of course you could.

But if you're like me, you're tired of throwing away bunches of rotten cilantro. You might find it cumbersome to peel around all the knobs on the ginger root, and even more so when it's fibers clog your juicer. You might want to use lemongrass in your cooking, but can't find it anywhere. Perhaps you're already an avid essential oils user, but are scared to cook with your oils because you just don't know how. You love them so much, you believe in their power, and you want to start ingesting them in more FUN and DELICIOUS ways!

These are the reasons why I wanted to learn how to effectively cook with essential oils. And when I set out on my search for healthy recipes that fit my plant-based vegan lifestyle, I couldn't find very many that I was excited about. And so this book was born, or at least the seed was planted for me to begin the recipe writing process.

Each culinary essential oil that is featured in this book, is celebrated with recipes that highlight the flavor that each imparts. Categorized by oil family, you'll also find ideas for how else you might use essential oils to tackle all sorts of health challenges. You've got them in your home already, you might as well start to use them in the most well-loved room in the house—your kitchen!

What to know before you get cooking

Cooking with essential oils is so convenient because it takes far less of an essential oil to flavor your food than if you were using dry seasonings, spices, or flavoring agents. Often even a single drop of an essential oil can be too overpowering, especially with the strong oils, so even the tiniest amount can add a serious blast of flavor to your dish.

In some recipes, it is appropriate to add an entire drop of essential oil but remember: once a drop has been added you cannot take it back. You can always add more to the dish if needed, so the toothpick method is recommended until you feel more comfortable cooking with essential oils.

The amount of essential oil added to a recipe depends largely on what kind of oil you are using, your personal taste preferences, and whether you are substituting the oil for raw, fresh, or dried ingredients. There are some guidelines that will help as you experiment with and enjoy cooking using essential oils.

It is best to add the essential oil toward the end of the recipe because the heat may lessen the efficacy and potency of the oil. The less time the oil is exposed to heat, the more flavor it will retain. If your recipe requires that you bake, steam, simmer, or boil, and you cannot add the essential oil at the end, simply add a larger amount of the oil, as some of the flavor will cook off. When cooking with strong oils like Oregano or Basil, it can be a good idea to let the oil simmer or evaporate to result in a milder, more pleasant flavor.

Use cookware and containers that are stainless steel, ceramic, or glass when cooking and mixing with essential oils because they can potentially damage some types of plastic. The flavor of the essential oil will strengthen overtime. So if preparing a dish ahead of time, add the oils just before serving to your family or guests.

Dilute in a Culinary Carrier Oil

Adding essential oils to a culinary carrier oil such as extra-virgin olive oil, avocado oil, hemp oil, flax oil, or grapeseed oil, etc is one of the best ways to flavor your dishes without overdoing it. Pour the carrier oil into a glass or metal dish and add the essential oils, the amount will vary depending on the essential oil used and the amount of carrier oil you are infusing. Once the oils are combined, drizzle it over your dish and enjoy the incredible flavor!

Mix into Good Quality Salt

Using salt as a medium to add essential oils to my recipes was such a game changer! By adding a few drops of essential oils to a few tablespoons of good quality salt, such as pink Himalayan or grey Celtic salt, you will be able to add potent flavor to your food, without adding much salt—it's a win-win! In this book you'll find many recipes for essential oil seasoning salts. Join me on social media **@cheflaurendagostino** to be among the first to know when I release my culinary make and take kit featuring these unique and flavorful salt blends!

Quick Kitchen Reference Guide

Hungry for an easy way to keep the basics handy as you get to cooking in your kitchen with essential oils? Download my Quick Kitchen Reference Guide as a free bonus for purchasing this cookbook at **www.laurendagostino.com/eo-cookbook.**

The Toothpick Method

Using the toothpick method when you are starting out, or when handling potent oils like oregano or cinnamon bark, is a good idea. To extract a small amount of oil from the bottle, simply insert a clean toothpick into the center orifice, it will only go about one third of the way into the bottle. Swirl the toothpick into the dish you are infusing the essential oil into, such as a soup, frosting, or marinade. If a stronger flavor is desired, repeat the process with a clean toothpick each time, until you're happy with the flavor. This requires tasting as you go, which I highly recommend forming a habit around if you're not there already. The taste should never be a mystery when you sit down to eat!

Final Thoughts

Learning how to trust yourself in the kitchen while preparing meals is one of the most liberating things we can experience. I still reach for recipes and cookbooks for inspiration from time to time, but with a little practice, you won't need to measure every single ingredient.

Remember that the recipes and ideas in this book are a starting place. What's listed is what works for me and my family, so if there is an ingredient that you don't care for or have access to, simply leave it out. If you get an idea to add something to any of the recipes, I encourage you to do so!

You know your body best, despite what you may think. So trust your instincts and your taste buds, put on some good music, get the diffuser going, and have the most fun preparing your food and cooking with essential oils!

-Chef Lauren

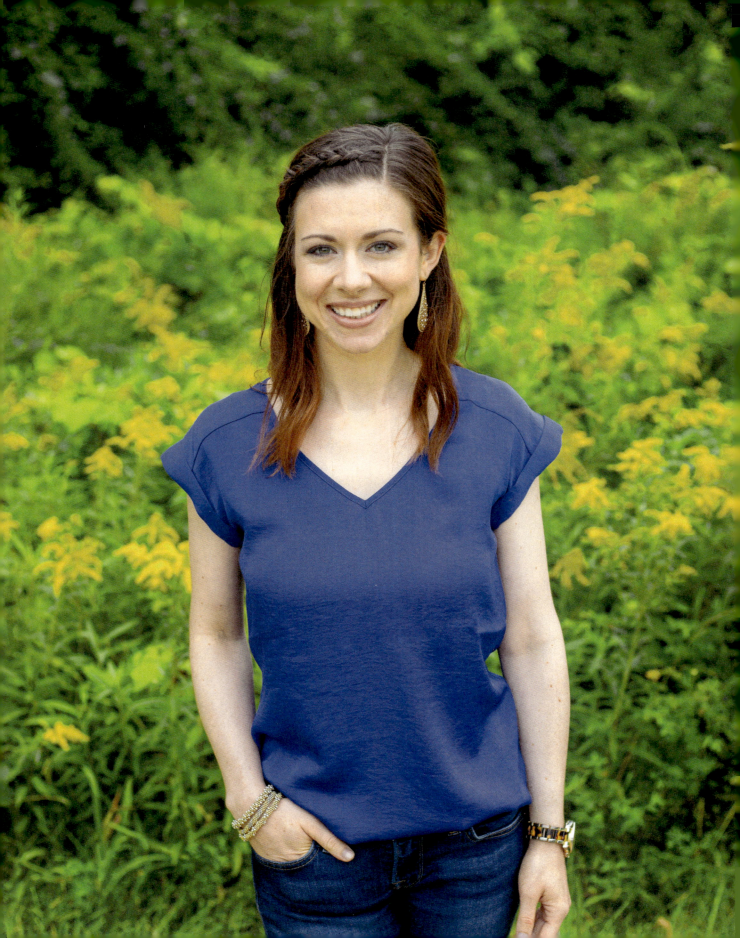

Chef Lauren's Story

From a young age, I always knew I wanted to be a chef, but I didn't always listen to my heart or believe in myself enough to jump all the way into the kitchen. After college, I worked in retail, managing a department store but after a few years I felt very unfulfilled and realized that it was time to fulfill a childhood dream and go to culinary school.

After attending Le Cordon Bleu's Patisserie and Baking Program in Cambridge, Massachusetts, I landed an opportunity to work at Disney World. After moving to Florida and working in the high-volume hotel industry, I began to question the work that I was doing. I still enjoyed making pastries and sweets, but I started to feel guilty about the lack of nutrition of these foods. I became bothered by the large amounts of dairy, eggs, and sugar, so I started to do some research of my own.

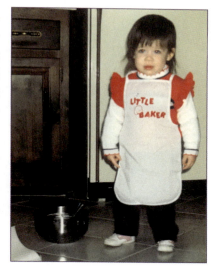

Working for Whole Foods Market as a cake decorator shortly after leaving Disney helped to open my eyes to a better way of eating. I had worked for the company while I was in pastry school as well, so the familiarity was appreciated in a place that still didn't feel like home. It was during this time that I became vegan again and really embraced the nutritional side of food and cooking.

A giant leap forward in the learning process was a position I held as a plant-based chef for a local juice bar, called Press'd, in Winter Garden, Florida. I discovered so much about plant-based cooking, but most importantly, how easy and delicious it could be! My world was changed, and I was loving all the new tastes. As much as I enjoyed working for Press'd Juice Bar and Kitchen, I decided it was time to head back to Massachusetts and figure out what was next. I transferred with Whole Foods into a position that gave me a break from production in the kitchen, and that was the beginning of a decline into an identity crisis.

I was bored.

I also lacked friendships and was living (with my boyfriend) at my parent's house—not an ideal situation! As I think about this time in my life now, it was a rock bottom that I desperately needed to shake me out of my comfort zone and discover a sense of purpose again. I searched high and low for what that might be and stumbled upon the Health Coach Training Program offered by the Institute for Integrative Nutrition (IIN).

This holistic health coach training program gave new meaning to my life—I was so fascinated by what I was learning about food and health. I appreciated the holistic approach to nutrition, especially since embracing a vegan diet years prior and evolving into more of the person I knew I wanted to be.

My intention, when I was ready to commit to a lifestyle change, was to fully embody a vegan, plant-based lifestyle that was in sync with the cycles of the seasons.

This included food, of course, but also other lifestyle components such as essential oils, astrology, and universal energy. I knew that all of these components of a holistic lifestyle were important for me to feel a deeper connection and sense of fulfillment that I'd been searching for ever since being asked the question, "What do you want to be when you grow up?"

This journey began with the food because I felt comfortable and capable in this arena, and because I believe that food is the foundation of everything that we are. It took a conscious effort to reevaluate my diet and actively choose what made sense for me each step of the way. I reset my mind to be patient and kind during this process and valued this commitment and connection to my intention. This was critical, and at times not easy, because I was working long days as a pastry chef and restaurant server at the time, constantly surrounded by temptation.

It took me about three months to achieve the lifestyle I wanted, and I've been able to sustain it for over four years. The first step for me was to eliminate red meat, which felt very doable because I never cared much for it anyway. I got comfortable in a lifestyle that did not include any red meat or meat products. When I went grocery shopping, I simply skipped over this section and my bill reduced. When I went out to eat, I had an easier time making decisions, something that had always been difficult for me, because I knew right away which items were not a fit for my lifestyle, thereby reducing my options. I lived within this dietary framework until red meat became something that I did not miss, did not crave, and did not think about.

The next step was to remove chicken and all other meat, which was slightly more challenging, though not difficult because I held that intention I had set so close to my awareness every single day. I thought about everything I had learned about the poor quality of the food group I was working to eliminate and what happened in my body when I consumed them. I learned to love fresh vegetables and salads and enjoyed stepping into a vegetarian lifestyle again. The pros were beginning to outweigh the cons and I was discovering so many new foods and cuisines that it was *exciting*, rather than limiting. I lived within this dietary framework until all meat and poultry became something that I did not miss, did not crave, and did not think about.

Becoming a full-time vegetarian by eliminating fish was a breeze after that because I had already fallen so in love with fruits and vegetables and had started to notice changes in my physical body. I was sleeping better, my skin was more radiant, my digestion improved, and I recovered faster in-between workouts. When I was cooking at home, preparation and clean-up had become so easy because I wasn't using any raw meat. Realizing that I could continue enjoying these benefits by also cutting out fish was a no brainer. When I went grocery shopping, my trips were faster because I had less retail space to explore. I discovered some amazing produce markets, farm stands, and other local vendors at farmers' markets. When I was dining out, I knew to look right for the vegetarian section. I had become more comfortable and confident when asking for what I wanted when modifications were required to meet my needs. I lived within this dietary framework until being vegetarian was something that I could own, something that I enjoyed, and something that I had become very good at.

A few months later, I took a big step in my journey by removing the dairy and eggs from my diet, which for many people is the hardest part, myself included. When I was making choices at the market and at home, I avoided these ingredients because it was easy to simply not buy them. When I was dining out, I still chose the vegetarian option and if dairy and eggs were part of the dish, I was forgiving of myself and found that I wasn't yet comfortable requesting a change to a menu item. I hadn't fully stepped into my ownership of a vegan plant-based diet and this decision to be kind with myself was a personal choice that really helped me lean into this new way of eating and living.

Once I started to see the difference in my skin and energy, I knew that I had to be a full-time plant-based vegan, but by then I was ready, and I knew why this was so important to me. I could really feel the affect it was having, and I was lucky to live in an area that had a large vegetarian and vegan community. It was then that I felt comfortable sharing my diet with people who asked, but before this point, I had kept it my business—because it was.

When you change your diet, it is important to stay focused on your intentions and the reasons for the change, without listening to outside influence or broadcasting your new lifestyle to friends and family who will try to take you off track. I know how hard it can be to keep information about how our food

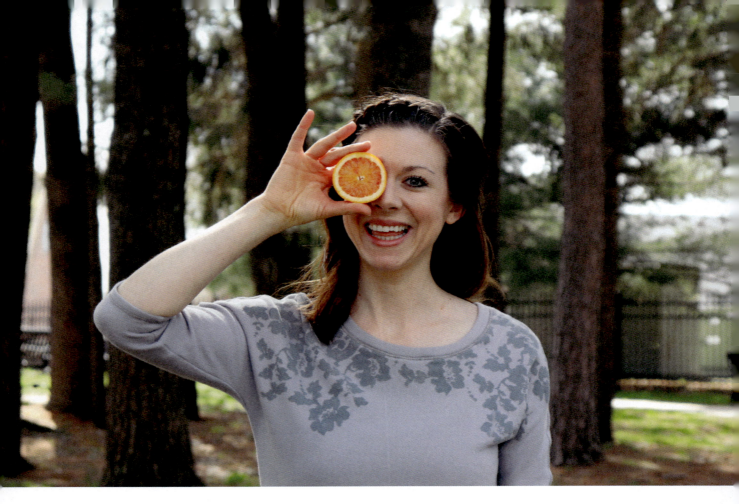

choices impact our health to ourselves, especially after watching any of the food and health films that are available for streaming. When I was able to lead by example instead of preach my diet to anyone with ears, I had an easier time sharing what I'd learned and what I'd been practicing because people were genuinely interested and wanted to know my secrets. Once I understood that every single body is different, I came to appreciate everyone's individual journey and started to become very curious about other people's reasons for becoming vegan.

The transition to living plant-based should be full of new discoveries for your taste buds and your body. You can eat whatever you like, but you will find over time that you will actively choose the healthier options, because intuitively it feels right. I still reach for recipes and cookbooks for inspiration from time to time, but with a little practice, you won't need to measure every single ingredient. You won't need to keep going back to the top of the recipe because you lost your place, again, and fear that you'll skip a step.

My hope for you is that you'll embrace the plant-based recipes and information in this book with an open mind and an empty belly, eager to taste the flavors of the earth. That you'll reconsider your food choices, because you are curious to experience a better quality of life. And that you'll discover the pure and potent flavor that essential oils can bring to your cooking, and to your life.

About the Author

Lauren D'Agostino is a private plant-based, vegan/gluten-free chef, intuitive cooking coach, and speaker sharing simple strategies for fast + flavorful plant-based cooking. She teaches clients her signature intuitive cooking methods to encourage and support cooks of any level in the first few steps of their transition to a plant-based diet.

Inspired by Ayurveda and her work as a professional vegan chef, the global consciousness shift, and her own transition into living a plant-based life, she is guiding others to create lasting habits by incorporating more plants, both on and off the plate.

She believes that everyone could benefit from eating and using more plants and works with her clients to teach them new strategies for plant-based meal preparation and healthcare. She shares her meal prep tips and cooking style with others in fun and engaging classes, workshops, and private instruction in home kitchens in New England and abroad.

She is a graduate of the Institute for Integrative Nutrition, the Isenberg School of Business at the University of Massachusetts Amherst, and the Patisserie & Baking Program at Le Cordon Bleu.

Connect with Lauren~

www.laurendagostino.com
www.facebook.com/cheflaurendagostino
my.doterra.com/cheflaurendagostino

KEY
T = Tablespoon   t = teaspoon

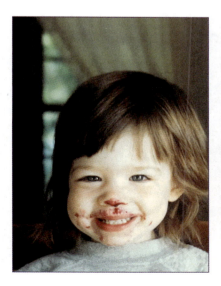
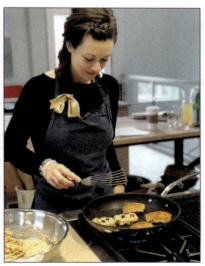
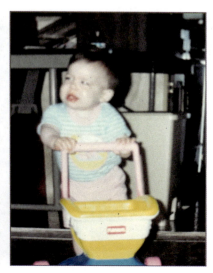

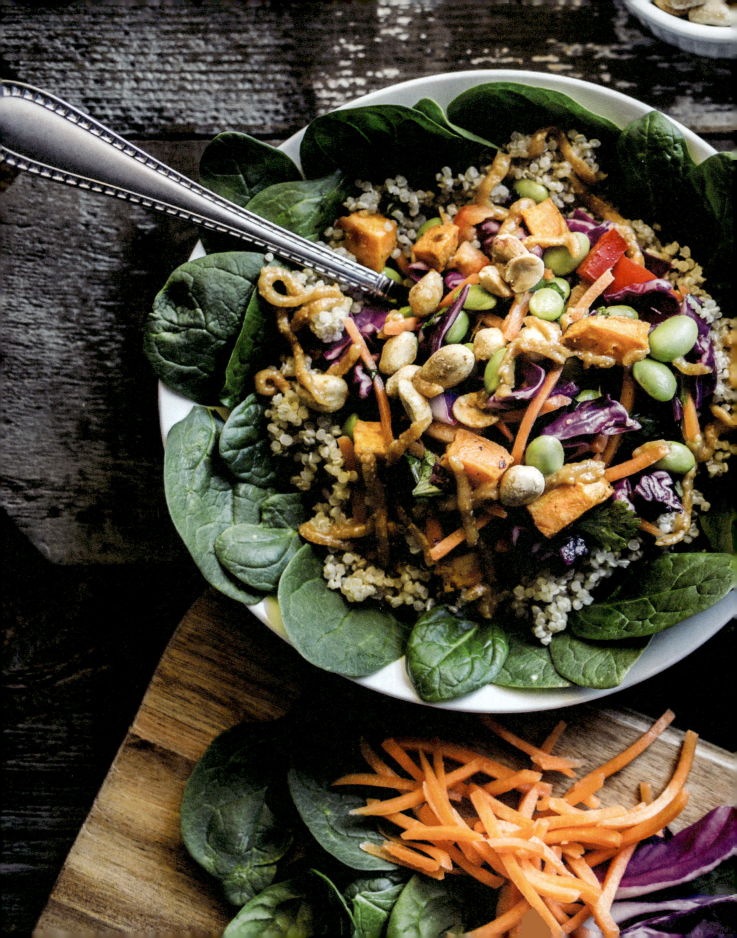

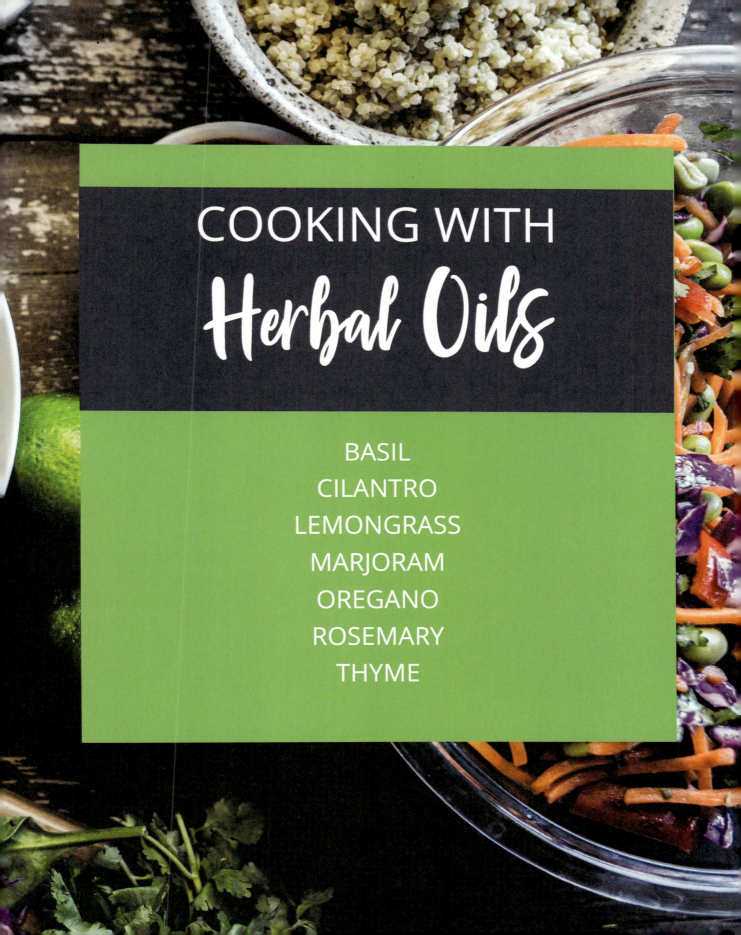

COOKING WITH
Herbal Oils

BASIL
CILANTRO
LEMONGRASS
MARJORAM
OREGANO
ROSEMARY
THYME

Top Uses for Herbal Essential Oils

Herbal oils provide a ton of amazing flavor, but they're also versatile and can be used to treat a variety of common conditions and ailments.

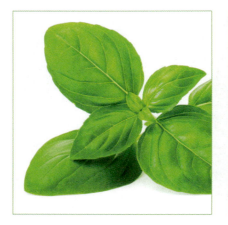

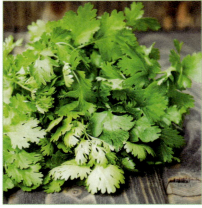

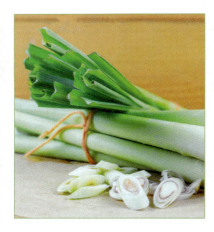

Basil

Adrenal fatigue, earache, loss of sense of smell, migraines, dizziness, mental fatigue, focus, nausea, cramping, gout, rheumatism, PMS, menstrual issues, emotional balance, muscle spasms, inflammation, snake, spider, bug bites

Cilantro

Heavy metal detox, gas, bloating, constipation, allergies, liver and kidney support, fungal and bacterial infections, body odor, anxiety, emotional balance

Lemongrass

Heavy metal detox, gas, bloating, constipation, allergies, liver and kidney support, fungal and bacterial infections, body odor, anxiety, emotional balance

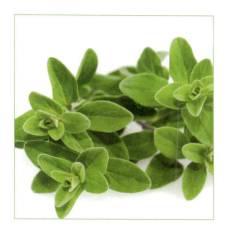

Marjoram

Carpal tunnel, tendinitis, arthritis, muscle cramps and sprains, high blood pressure and heart issues, croup and bronchitis, pancreatitis, overactive sex drive, boils, cold sores, ringworm, migraines and headaches, colic and constipation, calming and anxiety, emotional balance

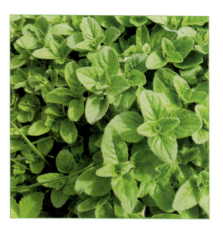

Oregano

Viruses and bacterial infections, strep throat and tonsillitis, staph infection and MRSA, intestinal worms and parasites, warts, calluses, canker sores, pneumonia and tuberculosis, boost progesterone, urinary infection, athlete's foot, ringworm, candida, carpal tunnel, rheumatism, emotional balance

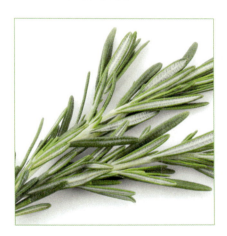

Rosemary

Respiratory infections and conditions, prostate issues and nighttime urination, cancer, hair loss and dandruff, memory and focus, bells' palsy and MS, mental, adrenal, and chronic fatigue, jaundice, liver and kidney issues, nervousness, depression, addiction, dopamine issues, muscle and bone pain, cellulite, jet lag, fainting, emotional balance

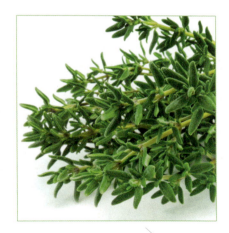

Thyme

Cold, flu and viruses, asthma, croup and pneumonia, candida and parasites, infertility, progesterone, breast, ovary and prostate issues, memory, concentration and dementia, low blood pressure, incontinence and bladder infection, fibroids and cancer, pain and sore muscles, fatigue, stress and depression, hair loss, emotional balance

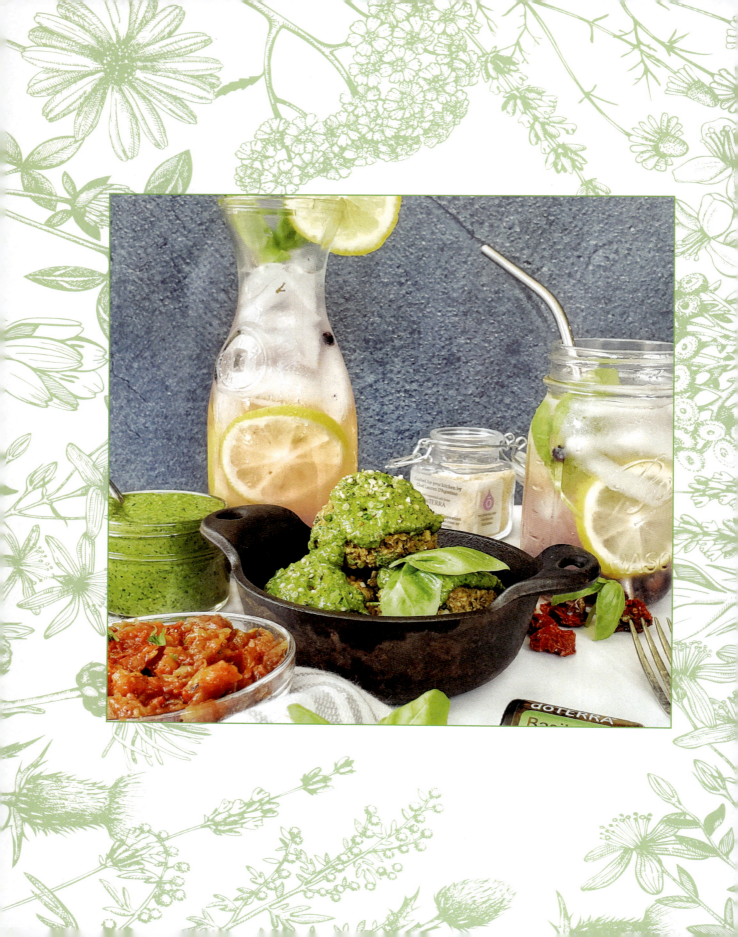

AROMA: SPICY + HERBAL | **FLAVORS:** SWEET + TENDER
PAIRS WITH: ITALIAN, CITRUS | **MAIN USES:** FOCUS + ALERTNESS

Basil

GREENS PESTO

1 cup baby spinach
1 cup baby kale
1 cup arugula
1/4 cup nutritional yeast
Salt and pepper
1/2 cup walnuts or pine nuts

1. Place all ingredients in a food processor and turn on to start blending.
2. Drizzle 1/4 cup good quality extra virgin olive oil until all incorporated and smooth.
3. Add 1 drop Basil essential oil and pulse 5 seconds to combine before transferring to storage container.

ITALIAN SEASONING SALT

3 T Himalayan pink salt
1 drop each Basil, Oregano, Thyme, Rosemary essential oils
1 T granulated garlic

Mix all in small jar with lid. Stir before using, a little goes a long way!

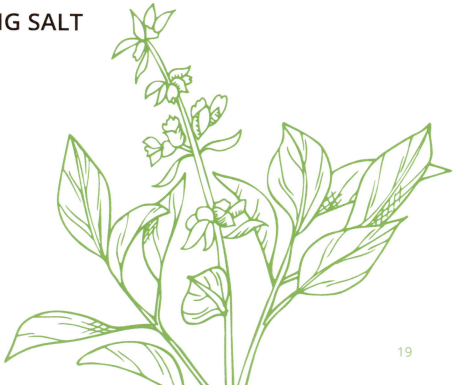

ROASTED TOMATO AND CARAMELIZED ONION SPREAD

1-2 yellow onions, diced
1-2 t white wine vinegar
1-2 pints cherry tomatoes

1. Sauté onions in pan over medium-low heat until onions are golden brown. Deglaze the pan with vinegar or regular white wine before adding tomatoes.
2. Add tomatoes and cook until popped. Add 1/4 t tapioca starch, arrowroot, or cornstarch to help thicken if needed. Season to taste with Italian seasoning salt.

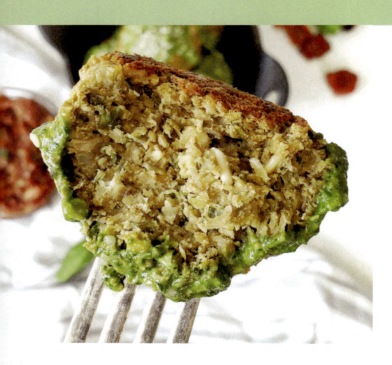

VEGAN LENTIL MEATBALLS

1 yellow onion, minced

3 cloves garlic, pressed
1 T flaxmeal
2 1/2 T water

1 1/2 cups cooked and cooled green lentils
1/2 t Italian seasoning salt
1/4 cup nutritional yeast
1 T tomato paste
1/4 cup parsley
1/2 cup oat flour

1. Saute onions over medium heat for 3-4 minutes, then add garlic and cook additional minute before removing from heat. Set aside.
2. Combine flaxmeal and water in a small bowl and let sit 5 minutes to form flax egg.
3. Mix all ingredients in a food processor, adding oat flour or coconut flour if too wet. Mixture should hold its shape when portioned into balls.
4. Portion and shape into balls and bake on lightly sprayed baking pan at 350°F for 20 minutes or until set and golden.
5. Serve with Greens Pesto and Tomato Jam.

BLUEBERRY BASIL LEMONADE

1/4 cup blueberries
2 T coconut sugar
12 oz Sparkling or still water
1 lemon, juiced
1 drop Lemon essential oil
Toothpick of Basil essential oil

1. Muddle blueberries in a glass with coconut sugar.
2. Add a splash of hot water to help dissolve the sugar before adding the lemon juice and water to the glass.
3. Garnish with lemon slices, a few blueberries, and fresh basil.

Basil essential oil is more floral than its fresh or dried form, so try to use it in recipes where heat is applied, or use the toothpick method so as not to add too much.

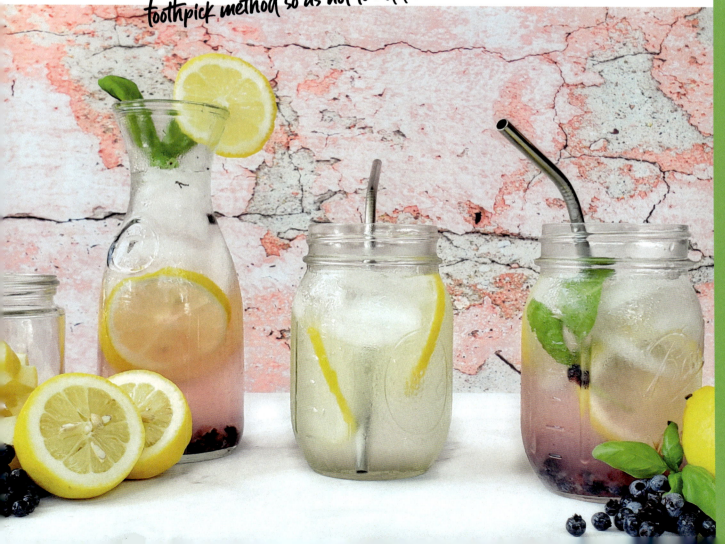

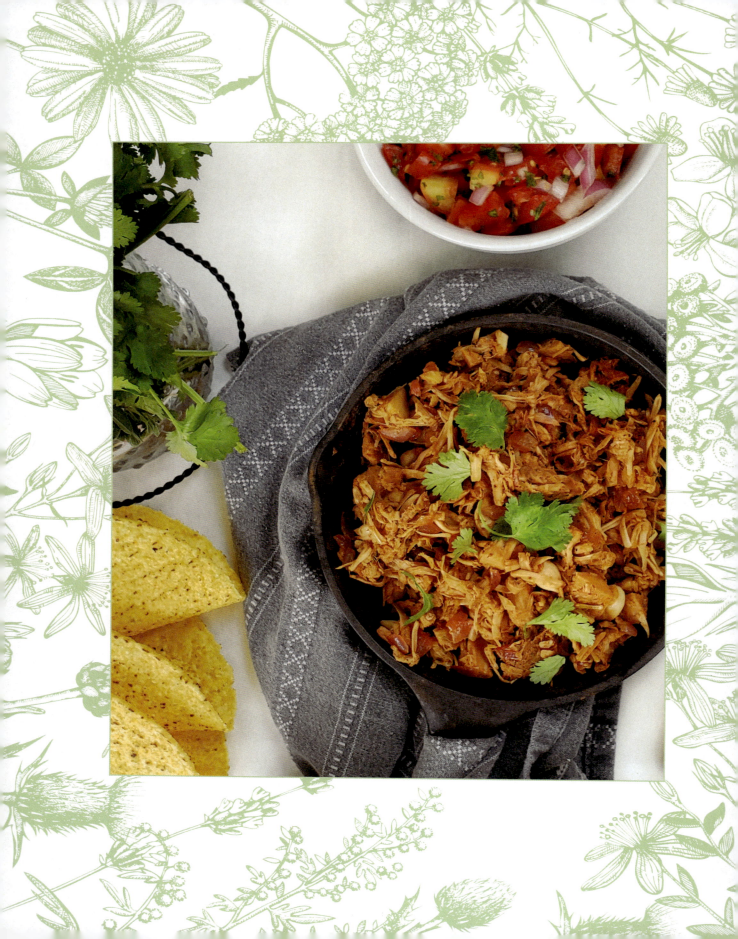

AROMA: HERBAL + PUNGENT | *FLAVORS:* REFRESHING
PAIRS WITH: CITRUS + GARLIC | *MAIN USES:* PURIFYING

Cilantro

PICO DE GALLO

2 tomatoes, diced
1/4 cup diced red onion
1/4 t fresh lime juice
pinch salt
1 drop Cilantro essential oil

Mix all ingredients in a bowl and enjoy with chips or as a condiment on tacos, power bowls, or salad.

MEXICAN SEASONING SALT

3 T Himalayan pink salt
1 drop each Cilantro, Lime, Coriander essential oils
1 T granulated garlic
1 T cumin

Mix all in small jar with lid. Stir before using, a little goes a long way!

CILANTRO LIME DRESSING

1/2 cup orange juice
1 cup spinach or baby kale
1 cup parsley
1/4 cup apple cider vinegar
1 drop each Cilantro and Lime essential oils
pinch xanthan gum

Blend all but the oils in a high-power blender until smooth. add oils in at the very end, pulse to combine. Enjoy this detoxifying dressing on salads, bowls, or as a marinade!

Learn to cook without measuring—it is so freeing to be able to use your judgment as you cook! And taste as you go, adjusting as needed.

FRESH GUACAMOLE

Avocados
Lime juice
Mexican seasoning salt

Smash avocado in a bowl with a whisk, adding lime juice to prevent browning and Mexican seasoning salt to taste.

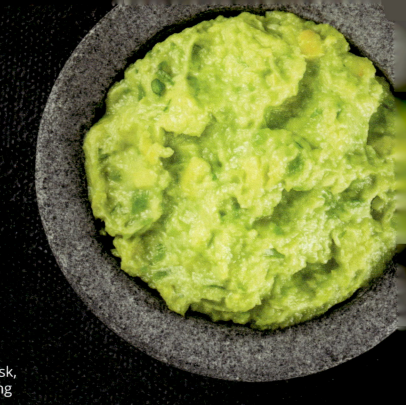

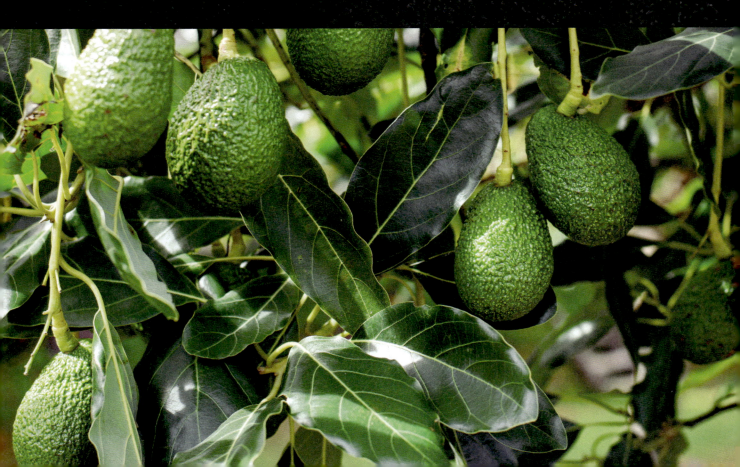

CARNITAS BRAISED JACKFRUIT

1 t avocado oil
1/2 yellow onion, diced
1 clove garlic, pressed

1 can jackfruit in brine or water, drained and rinsed

1 t cumin
1 t nutritional yeast
1 t oregano
1 t smoked paprika
1/4 t pepper
1/4 t salt
1 T coconut aminos
1 t apple cider vinegar
1 t orange juice

1 t lime juice
1 drop Cilantro essential oil

1. Saute onion and garlic in the avocado oil, in a medium size pan, over medium heat until fragrant—about 4 minutes.
2. Add rinsed jackfruit, breaking up the pieces as needed.
3. Add all ingredients, up to orange juice, to the pan to continue cooking, covered, on medium low heat. Cook about 8 minutes—until the jackfruit is soft and well coated with seasoning.
4. Remove from heat.
5. Squeeze lime juice into a small dish and add one drop of Cilantro essential oil—it is important to dilute the oil in a carrier for even flavor distribution.
6. Add lime juice to the jackfruit and use in tacos, on bowls, in quesadillas or to top nachos or a Mexican vegan pizza!

THAI SEASONING SALT

3 T Himalayan pink salt
1 drop each Cilantro, Lime, Lemongrass essential oils
1 T granulated garlic

Mix all in small jar with lid. Stir before using, a little goes a long way!

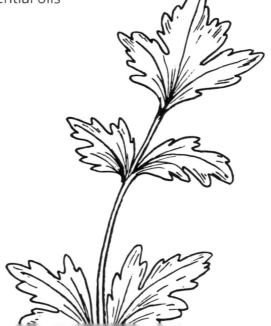

25

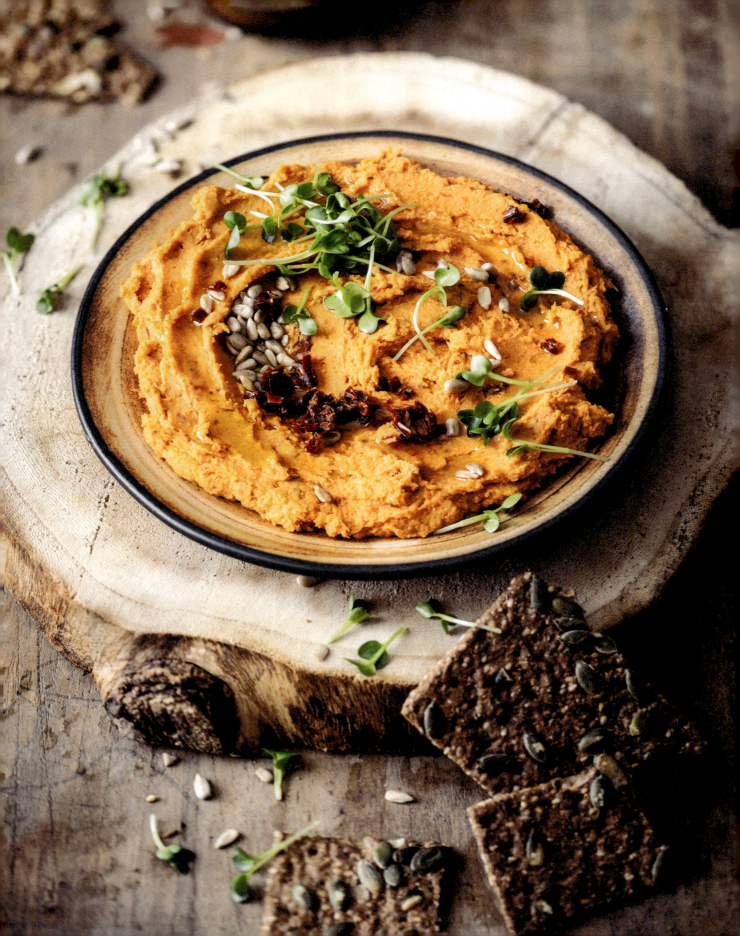

AROMA: *CITRUS + SMOKEY* | **FLAVORS:** *PUNGENT + FLORAL*
PAIRS WITH: *CURRY + COCONUT* | **MAIN USES:** *MASSAGE*

Lemongrass

THAI HUMMUS

2 15-oz cans chickpeas, drained and rinsed
2 T red curry paste
1 T tahini
1 t salt
1 T turmeric powder
1 t lemon juice
1 drop each Lemongrass, Cilantro, Ginger essential oils
1-2 T extra-virgin olive oil

1. Add all ingredients, except the essential oils, to the bowl of a food processor and mix well, scraping the sides as needed.
2. Add the oils in the last few seconds of blending so as not to disturb their integrity.

Make hummus a kitchen staple and add it to everything!

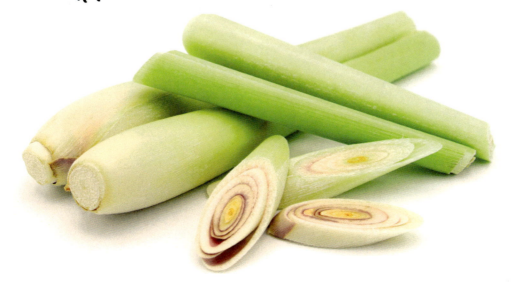

27

COCONUT GREEN CURRY BRAISED JACKFRUIT

2 T green curry paste (see recipe below)
1 can coconut milk
1 cup veggie stock
2 cans green jackfruit in water or brine, rinsed
Salt and pepper to taste

1. Combine ingredients in crock pot and set to low for 5-6 hours.
2. Enjoy over brown rice with wilted greens and seasonal veggies! Garnish with fresh cilantro and lime wedges.

Note: Can also be prepared in a saute pan over medium-low heat, covered, until jackfruit is soft and sauce is reduced, about 20 minutes.

GREEN CURRY PASTE

8-oz serrano chiles
1 medium yellow onion
4 cloves garlic
1 t salt
1 t coconut sugar
1 t turmeric powder
1 t coriander
1 t cumin
1 drop each Lemongrass and Ginger essential oils

1. Add all ingredients, except the essential oils, to the bowl of a food processor and mix well. Scrape down the sides as needed.
2. Add the essential oils in the last few seconds of blending.
3. Combine with coconut milk and season to taste for an easy Thai green curry!

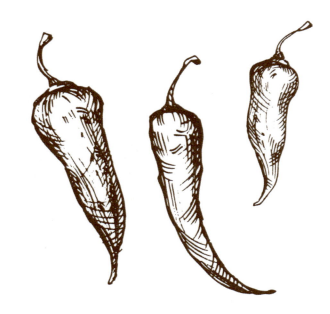

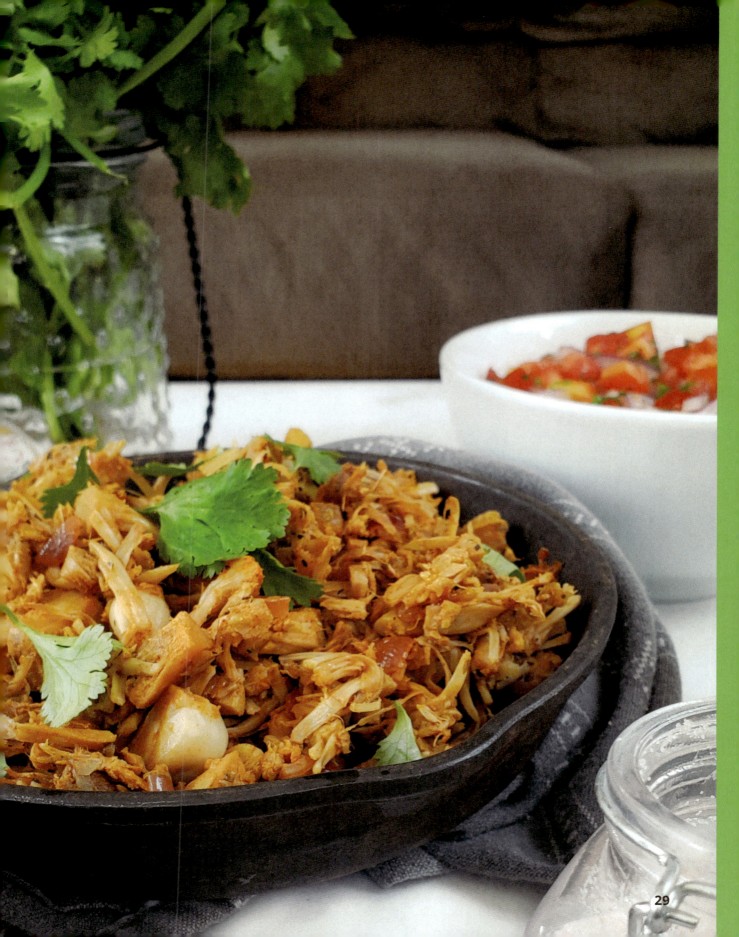

ADD LEMONGRASS TO YOUR STIR FRY!

1. Combine equal parts tamari and water in a dish with a little cornstarch and add 1 drop each Lemongrass, Ginger, and Lime essential oils.
2. Add mixture to the pan or wok at the end of stir frying and stir well to coat and reduce the sauce.

Note: Be careful not to cook the essential oils too long, as the flavor will cook off. I like to shut the heat off right after I add the sauce, continue stirring, and serve immediately.

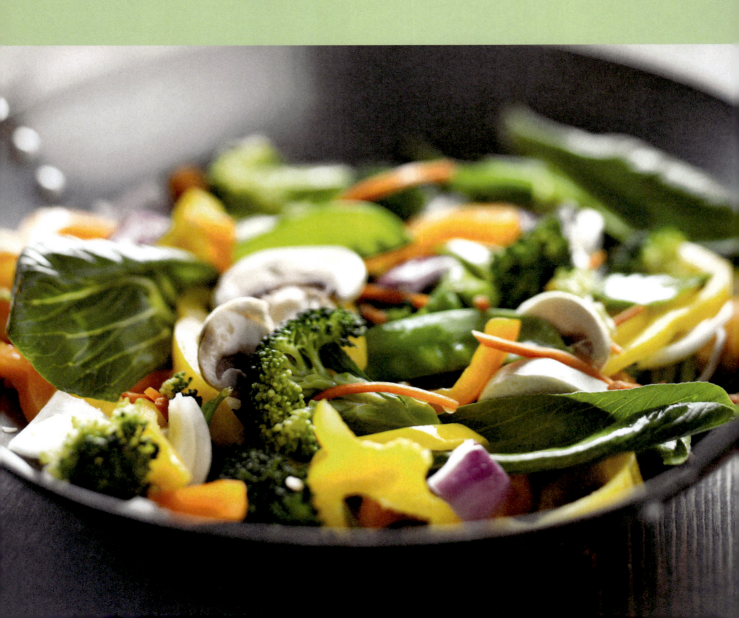

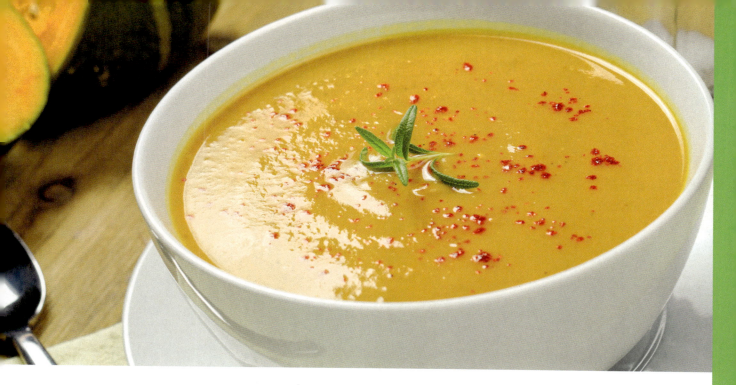

THAI BUTTERNUT SOUP

1 medium yellow onion, diced
2 cloves garlic, rubbed over microplane
4 cups vegetable broth
1 medium butternut squash, peeled and cubed
1 can coconut milk
2 T red curry paste
1 T turmeric powder
1 t cumin
salt and pepper to taste
1 drop each Lemongrass, Cilantro, Ginger essential oils

1. Saute the onion over medium heat until fragrant and soft, about 4 minutes.
2. Add fresh pressed or grated garlic, heat one minute.
3. Add all other ingredients, except essential oils. Cook on low, covered, until squash is tender.
4. Carefully blend in a high-powered blender or with an immersion blender. Add essential oils just before serving.

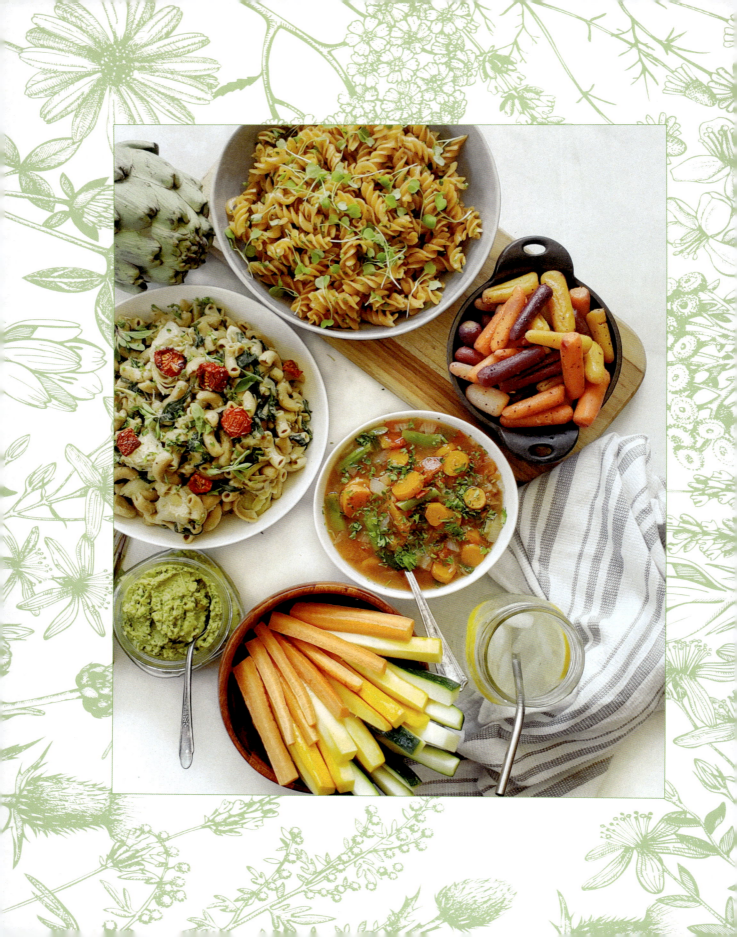

AROMA: *WARM + WOODY* | **FLAVORS:** *CITRUS + BRIGHT*
PAIRS WITH: *LEMON + TOMATO* | **MAIN USES:** *SOOTHING*

Marjoram

SPINACH ARTICHOKE HUMMUS

2 cans chickpeas or cannellini beans, drained and rinsed
1 clove fresh garlic, pressed
1 T tahini
1 can artichoke hearts, drained
1/2 bag frozen spinach, thawed
2 T nutritional yeast
1 tsp lemon juice

Salt and pepper to taste

Blend all ingredients in a food processor and drizzle in water/broth or olive/avocado oil until your preferred hummus texture is reached. Add 1 drop Marjoram essential oil in toward the very end of blending.

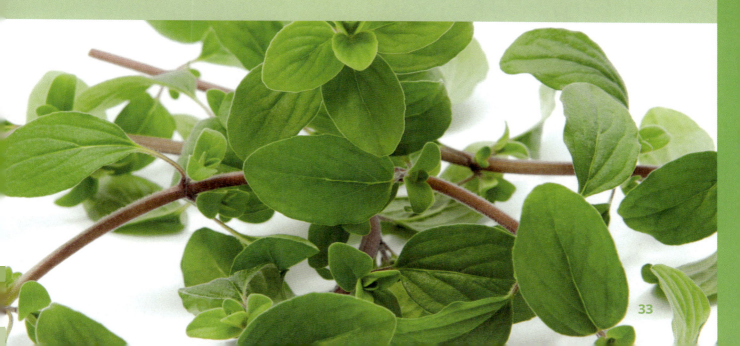

SPINACH ARTICHOKE PASTA

1 yellow onion, diced
1 clove fresh pressed garlic
1 t white wine vinegar

1 box GF pasta
2 cups water
1/2 cup nutritional yeast
1/4 t fresh cracked pepper

Handfuls of fresh spinach or kale
1 can artichoke hearts, drained and chopped

1. In a medium pot, saute the onion until fragrant—about 4 minutes.
2. Add garlic and cook for 1 minute more. Deglaze the pot with white wine vinegar, or regular white wine (something dry).
3. Add the pasta, water, nutritional yeast, and pepper to the pot. Stir to combine before turning up the heat to bring to a low boil.
4. Reduce heat to low and simmer, with a lid, until pasta is cooked—about 5 minutes.
5. Add tons of fresh spinach or baby kale and the artichokes. Continue cooking until greens are wilted and pasta is cooked.
6. Add one drop of Marjoram essential oil to a small dish with 1 T extra virgin olive oil, to dilute the flavor for even distribution.
7. Pour over pasta, season with salt to taste, and garnish with sun-dried tomatoes, fresh parsley, vegan parmesan.

HERBED PASTA

1 box GF pasta
1-2 T melted vegan butter or extra virgin olive oil
1 drop each Marjoram, Thyme, Rosemary essential oils
1 clove fresh pressed garlic

1. Cook pasta according to package directions.
2. In the serving bowl, combine oil or butter with essential oils and garlic.
3. Add cooked pasta and toss to coat.
4. Season to taste with pink salt and fresh cracked pepper.
5. Garnish with fresh parsley, toasted pine nuts, and vegan parmesan cheese.

QUICK SUMMER MINESTRONE SOUP

1-2 cloves garlic, pressed
1 onion, diced

3-4 cups summer vegetables:
   -zucchini/summer squash
   -beans
   -tomatoes
   -carrots
6 cups vegetable broth
1 can cannellini beans, drained
1 t salt
1/2 t pepper

1 drop each Thyme and Marjoram essential oils

1. Saute in a soup pot until fragrant, about 4 minutes. Add a splash of white wine vinegar to deglaze if needed.
2. Add chopped veggies of your choice—whatever grows locally makes the best soup!
3. Add broth, beans, and spices, then cover and cook over medium/low heat until vegetables are tender, about 15-20 minutes.
4. Add essential oils and remove soup from heat.

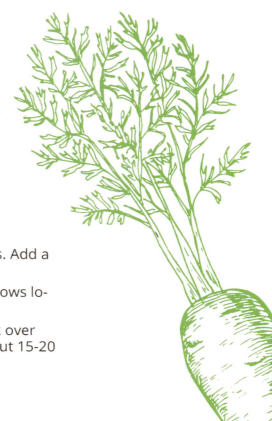

LEMON HERB CARROTS

1 bunch carrots, about 1 lb or 2 cups chopped

2 T melted vegan butter or extra virgin olive oil
1 drop Marjoram essential oil
1 t lemon juice
1 t maple syrup
Salt and pepper to taste

1. Cook carrots, organic and local if possible, however you like—sliced and sauteed, steamed baby, julienned or half mooned and roasted in a little avocado oil.
2. Add all other ingredients to a small dish to combine before pouring over cooked carrots. Season to taste and garnish with fresh herbs or toasted nuts.

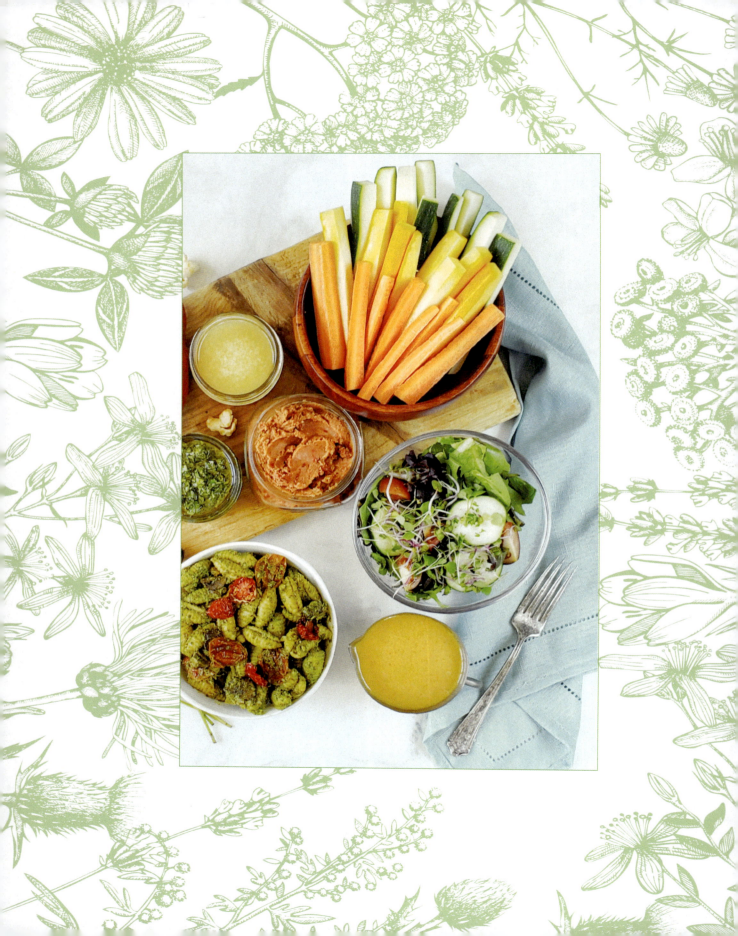

AROMA: SHARP + GREEN | ***FLAVORS:*** BITTER + PUNGENT
PAIRS WITH: MUSHROOM + TOMATO | ***MAIN USES:*** IMMUNITY

Oregano

EXPRESS PASTA SAUCE

2 cans fire roasted tomatoes, low sodium
1 tsp each garlic and onion powder
1 drop each Oregano, Thyme, Basil essential oils

Blend in a food processor until tomatoes are mostly blended. Warm sauce and toss with cooked pasta or roasted veggies, or use on pizza or as a dipping sauce!

HERBAL MARINADE

1/2 cup white wine vinegar
1 T lemon juice
1/4 cup avocado oil
1 clove fresh garlic, pressed
1 drop each Oregano, Rosemary, Thyme essential oils

Combine in a glass dish and add veggies or plant-based protein to marinade for several hours before cooking.

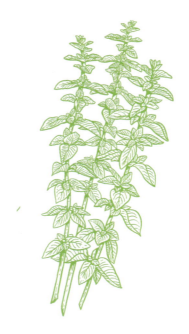

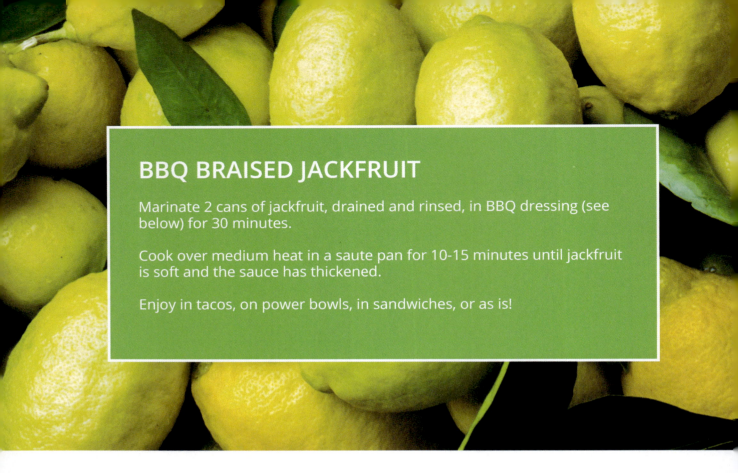

BBQ BRAISED JACKFRUIT

Marinate 2 cans of jackfruit, drained and rinsed, in BBQ dressing (see below) for 30 minutes.

Cook over medium heat in a saute pan for 10-15 minutes until jackfruit is soft and the sauce has thickened.

Enjoy in tacos, on power bowls, in sandwiches, or as is!

BBQ DRESSING

1 cup ketchup
1/4 cup apple cider vinegar
2 T molasses
2 T maple syrup
1 t Dijon mustard
1 t smoked paprika
1/2 t each garlic and onion powder
1 t liquid smoke
1/4 cup water
1/2 t sriracha
1/2 t chili powder
1 drop each Oregano and Basil essential oils

Blend all ingredients in blender, adding more water if thinner dressing is preferred.

GREEK DRESSING

1 cup red wine vinegar
1/2 cup extra virgin olive oil
1 T lemon juice
1/4 cup maple syrup
1/2 t garlic powder
1/4 cup Dijon mustard
1 drop Oregano essential oil

Blend all ingredients in a blender until a smooth emulsion is reached. Enjoy on salads, bowls, or as a marinade for your favorite veggies or tofu!

GREEK SEASONING SALT

3 T Himalayan pink salt
1 drop each Oregano and Lemon essential oils
1 T granulated garlic

Mix all in small jar with lid. Stir before using, a little goes a long way!

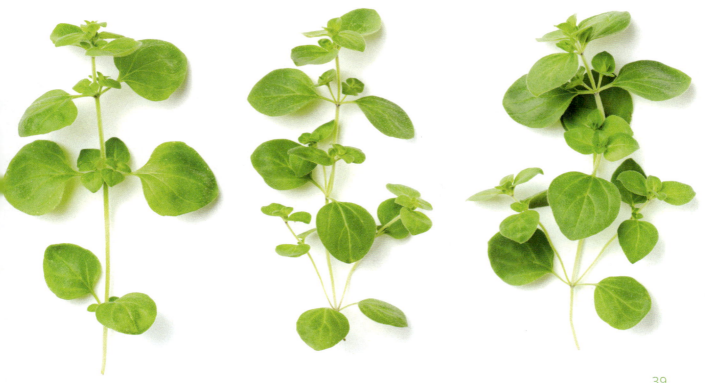

OREGANO PESTO

3 cups total spinach, baby kale, mixed greens, arugula, etc.
1/4 cup your favorite nut or seed
1 clove fresh grated garlic
1/4 cup nutritional yeast
1 drop each Lemon and Oregano essential oils

Blend all ingredients in a food processor until smooth. Drizzle in extra virgin olive oil 1 T at a time until desired consistency is reached. For pesto marinade, add 1/2 cup white wine vinegar or 1/3 cup apple cider vinegar.

CHIMICHURRI

1 cup parsley, finely chopped
1 clove fresh grated garlic
1/4 cup avocado oil
2 T white wine vinegar
2 T apple cider vinegar
Salt and pepper to taste
1 drop Oregano essential oil

Combine all ingredients in a bowl and use as a marinade for cauliflower steaks, roasted veggies, or tempeh.

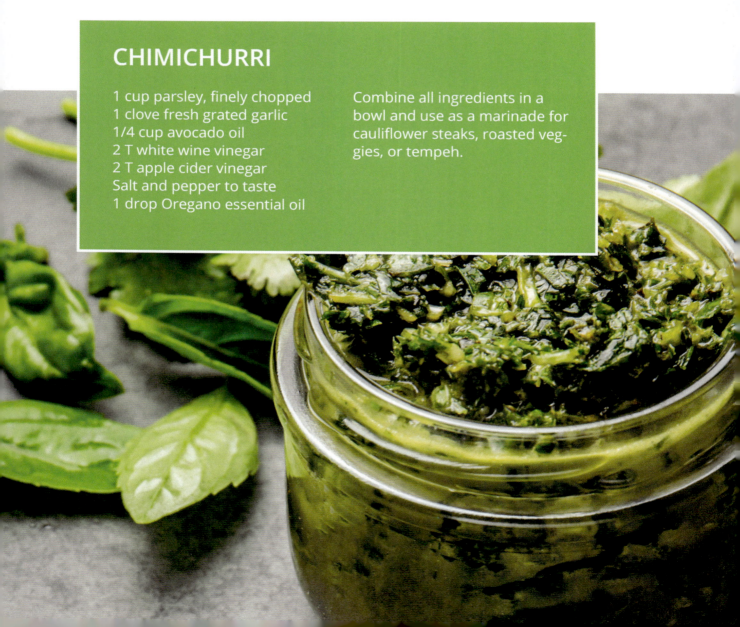

PIZZA POPCORN

1. Pop organic popcorn kernels in an air popper.
2. In a small bowl, add 3 T extra virgin olive oil and 1 drop each Oregano and Basil essential oils.
3. Toss with popcorn and sprinkle with Himalayan pink salt, black pepper, nutritional yeast, and smoked paprika for a little natural red color.

ROASTED GARLIC SPREAD

4 heads garlic
1 15 oz can cannellini beans, drained and rinsed
1/4 t salt
3 T avocado oil

1. Remove the outer skin from the garlic heads, leaving the cloves attached. Cut off the tops of the heads and place on a large sheet of foil, then drizzle with oil before wrapping and roasting at 400°F for one hour.
2. Once cool, remove cloves from the skin and place into a food processor. Puree until smooth, adding more oil as needed, and one drop of Oregano essential oil.

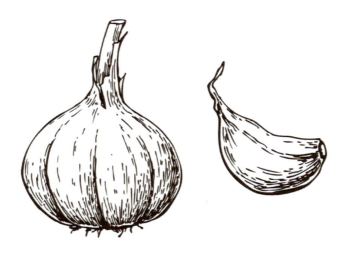

PASTA PRIMAVERA

1 yellow onion, diced
1 clove fresh pressed garlic
1 t white wine vinegar

1 box GF pasta
2 cups water
1/4 cup nutritional yeast
1/4 t fresh cracked pepper

Handfuls of fresh spinach or kale

Chopped spring or summer vegetables, such as cherry tomatoes, zucchini, summer squash, asparagus, green beans.

1. In a medium pot, saute the onion until fragrant—about 4 minutes.
2. Add garlic and cook for 1 minute more. Deglaze the pot with white wine vinegar, or regular white wine (something dry).
3. Add the pasta, water, nutritional yeast, and pepper to the pot. Stir to combine before turning up the heat to bring to a low boil.
4. Reduce heat to low and simmer, with a lid, until pasta is cooked—about 5 minutes.
5. Add tons of fresh spinach or baby kale and the chopped vegetables. Continue cooking until greens are wilted and pasta is cooked.
6. Add one drop of Oregano essential oil to a small dish with 1 T extra virgin olive oil, to dilute the flavor for even distribution.
7. Pour over pasta, season with salt to taste, and garnish with sun-dried tomatoes, fresh parsley, vegan parmesan cheese, or fresh cracked pepper.

Rosemary, Thyme, or Black Pepper essential oil are delicious substitutes for Oregano. Use spread with fresh veggies, on pizza, in bowls, in salad dressings, marinades, or soups!

SUN-DRIED TOMATO HUMMUS

2 cans chickpeas or cannellini beans, drained and rinsed
1 cup sun-dried tomatoes, soaked in hot water then drained
1 tsp lemon juice
1/4 t salt
1/4 t pepper
2 T broth or oil
1 drop Oregano essential oil

Blend all ingredients in a food processor and drizzle in water/broth or olive/avocado oil until your preferred hummus texture is reached. Add Oregano essential oil in toward the very end of blending.

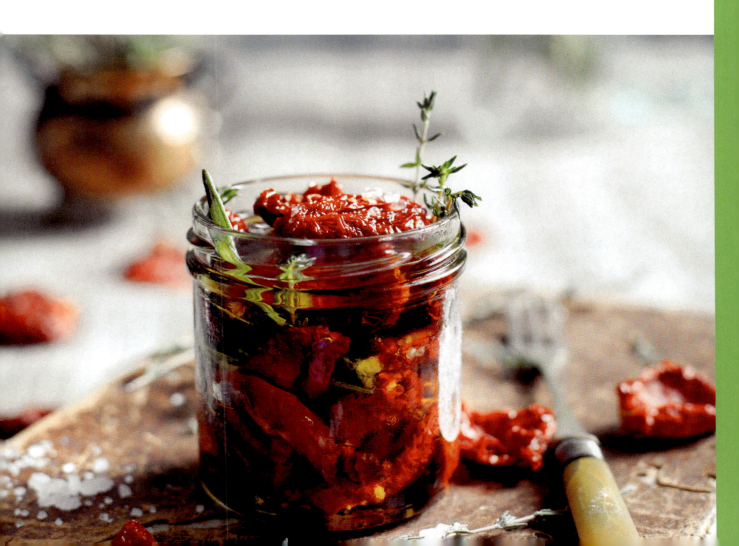

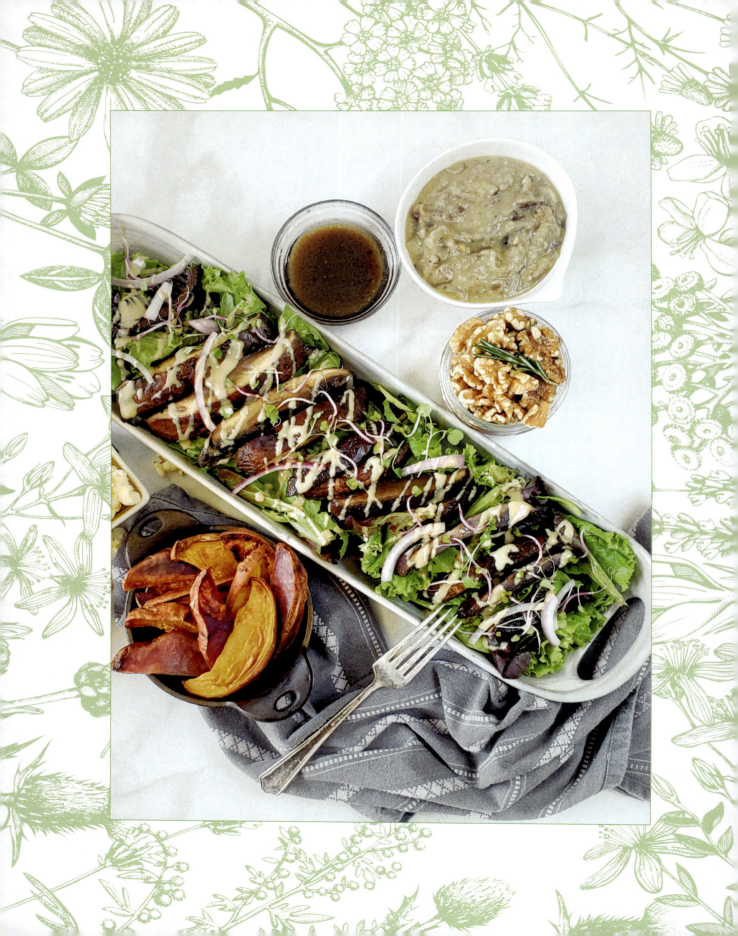

AROMA: *HERBACEOUS* | **FLAVORS:** *SHARP + WOODY*
PAIRS WITH: *MUSHROOMS* | **MAIN USES:** *RESPIRATORY*

Rosemary

ROSEMARY BALSAMIC MARINADE

1/4 cup balsamic vinegar
2 T avocado oil
2 drops Rosemary essential oil
1 clove fresh grated garlic

Combine all ingredients in a bowl before adding veggies.

Portobello mushroom caps, eggplant slices, and organic tofu work well.

Marinate overnight and roast or grill before adding to salad, bowls and more!

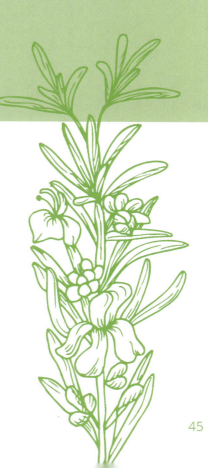

ROSEMARY ROASTED WALNUTS

2 cups walnuts
1/4 t avocado oil
2 drops Rosemary essential oil

1. Roast nuts plain at 250°F for 12-15 minutes.
2. Combine oils in bowl before adding nuts.
3. Season with salt to taste.

MUSHROOM GRAVY

1 onion, chopped
2 cloves fresh grated garlic

2 cups mushrooms, sliced or chopped

2 cups vegetable broth
2 t white miso
2 T gluten-free flour blend
1 T tamari, low sodium
1 T white wine vinegar

2 drops Rosemary essential oil

1. Cook chopped onion in a medium pot over medium heat until fragrant and soft, about 4 minutes.
2. Add fresh pressed garlic and cook one minute more. Deglaze the pan with white wine vinegar if needed.
3. Add mushrooms and cook until soft and slightly browned.
4. Whisk all other ingredients, except the essential oil, in a measuring cup before adding to the pot. Continue cooking over medium heat until flour has thickened the gravy to your liking.
5. Add essential oil and remove from heat.

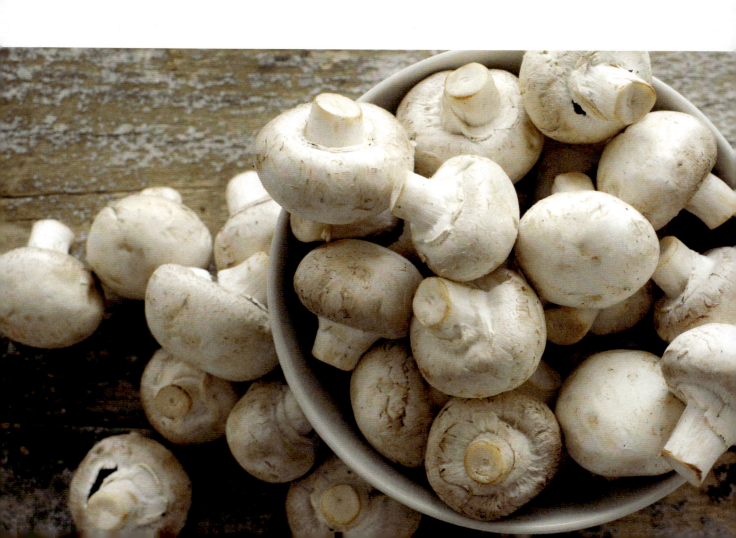

ROSEMARY ROASTED SWEET POTATOES

1 onion, diced
2-3 sweet potatoes, cut into wedges

Dressing:
1/2 t avocado oil
3 drops Rosemary essential oil
2 cloves fresh grated garlic
1/2 t salt
1/4 t pepper

Mix dressing ingredients in a medium bowl before adding potato and onion. Toss to coat and bake at 400°F for 15-20 minutes or until tender and crispy.

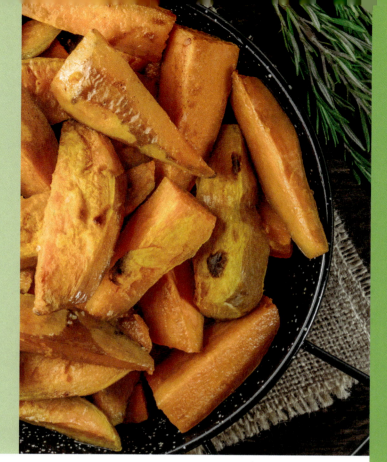

ROSEMARY POPCORN

Pop organic popcorn kernels in an air popper.

In a small bowl, add 3 T Extra virgin olive oil and 2 drops each Rosemary and Black Pepper essential oils.

Toss with popcorn and sprinkle with Himalayan pink salt and nutritional yeast.

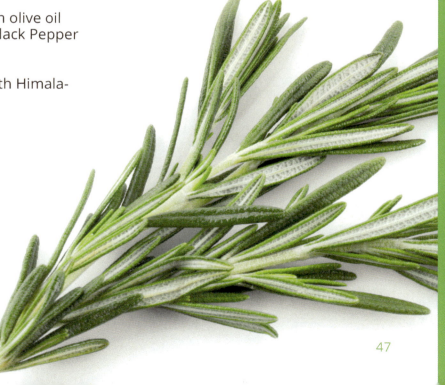

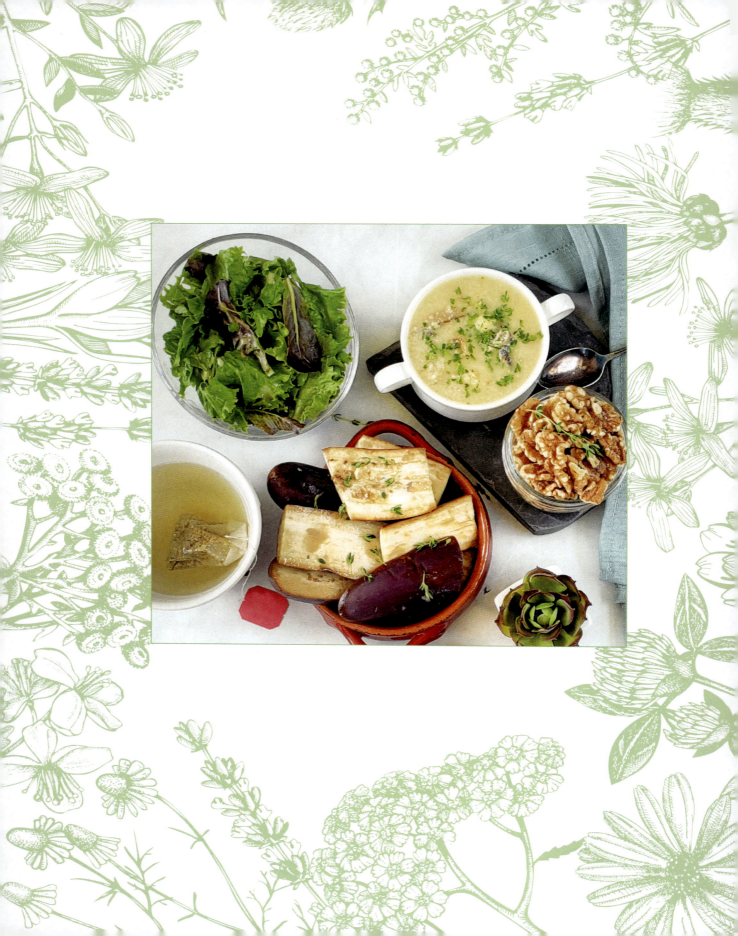

AROMA: *WARM + HERBACEOUS* | **FLAVORS:** *MINTY + EARTHY*
PAIRS WITH: *LEMON + TOMATO* | **MAIN USES:** *PURIFYING*

Thyme

ITALIAN MARINATED EGGPLANT

1/4 cup white wine vinegar
2 T avocado oil
2 drops Thyme essential oil
1 drop Marjoram essential oil
1 clove fresh grated garlic

1. Combine all ingredients in a bowl before adding eggplant slices. Marinate overnight and roast at 350°F or grill on medium-high heat before adding to salad, bowls and more.
2. Serve with express pasta sauce or pesto!

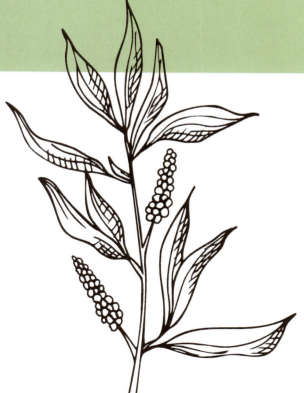

Vegetable broth seasoning can be found in health food stores in the soup aisle. I prefer to keep this on hand and make the broth fresh when I need it. Makes a great all purpose seasoning for veggie burgers too!

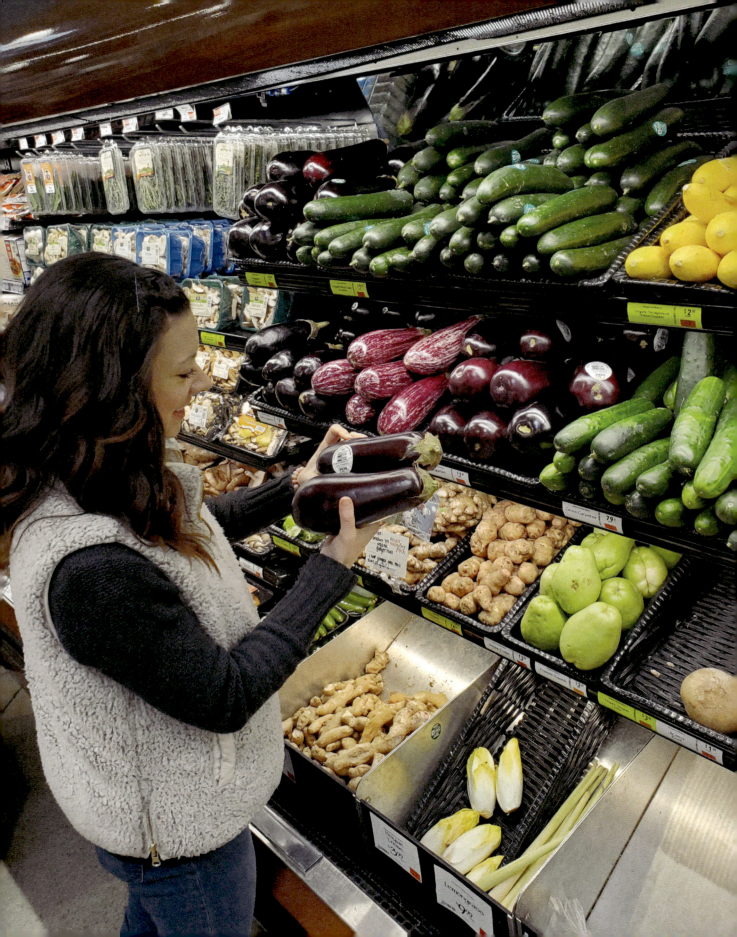

VEGAN CLAM CHOWDER

1 medium onion, diced
2 cloves garlic, grated/pressed
3 stalks celery, diced
1 T vegan butter

Clams:
1 cup shiitake mushrooms, chopped
2 T tamari
1 t liquid smoke
2 T kelp granules
1 T vegan butter

4 t vegetable broth seasoning
4 cups water
2 medium white potatoes, diced

1 drop Thyme essential oil
1/2 t salt
1/4 t black pepper

Cashew Cream:
1 cup cashews and 2 cups water in high powered blender until smooth.

1. Prepare mushroom clams first by adding the ingredients listed to a medium pan and cooking over medium heat until the mushrooms have softened and the liquid has cooked off or been absorbed.
2. Saute the onion, garlic, celery, and vegan butter in a soup pot on medium heat until fragrant, about 5 minutes.
3. Add the vegetable broth and potatoes to the pot and cook, covered, on medium/high heat until bubbling, then reduce heat to low and simmer until potatoes are soft.
4. Add the cashew cream and the mushroom clams. Heat the chowder through until bubbling and thick. Garnish with fresh parsley.

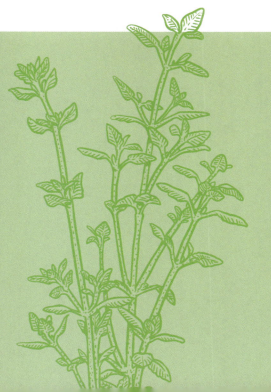

THYME ROASTED PINE NUTS

2 cups pine nuts
1 t avocado oil
1/4 t salt
2 drops Thyme essential oil

1. Roast nuts plain at 250°F for 5-7 minutes.
2. Combine oils in bowl before adding nuts. Season with salt to taste.

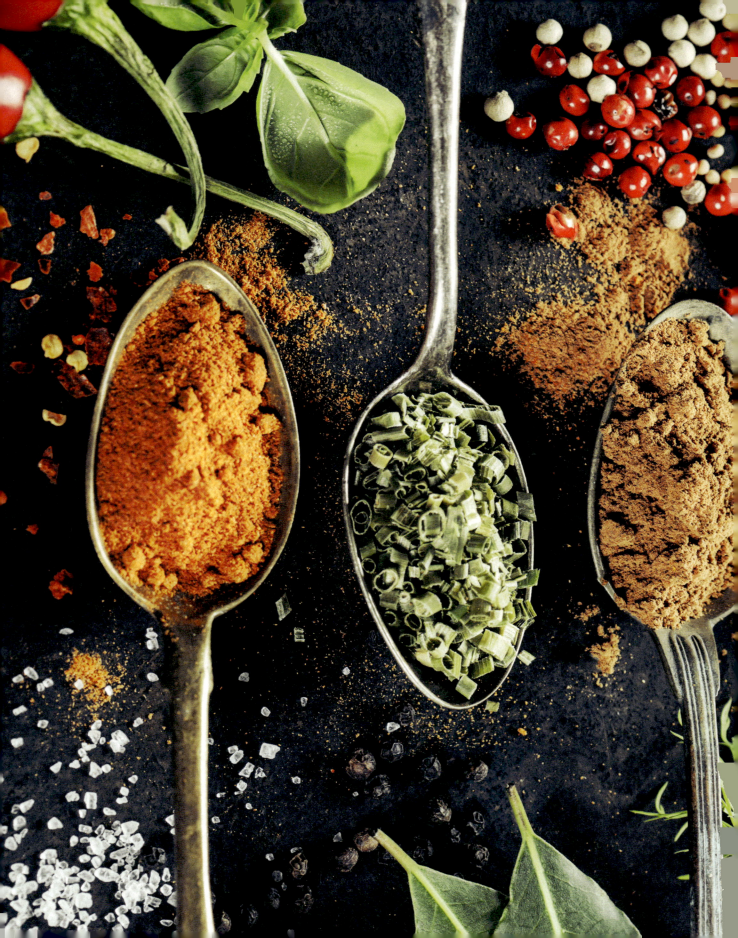

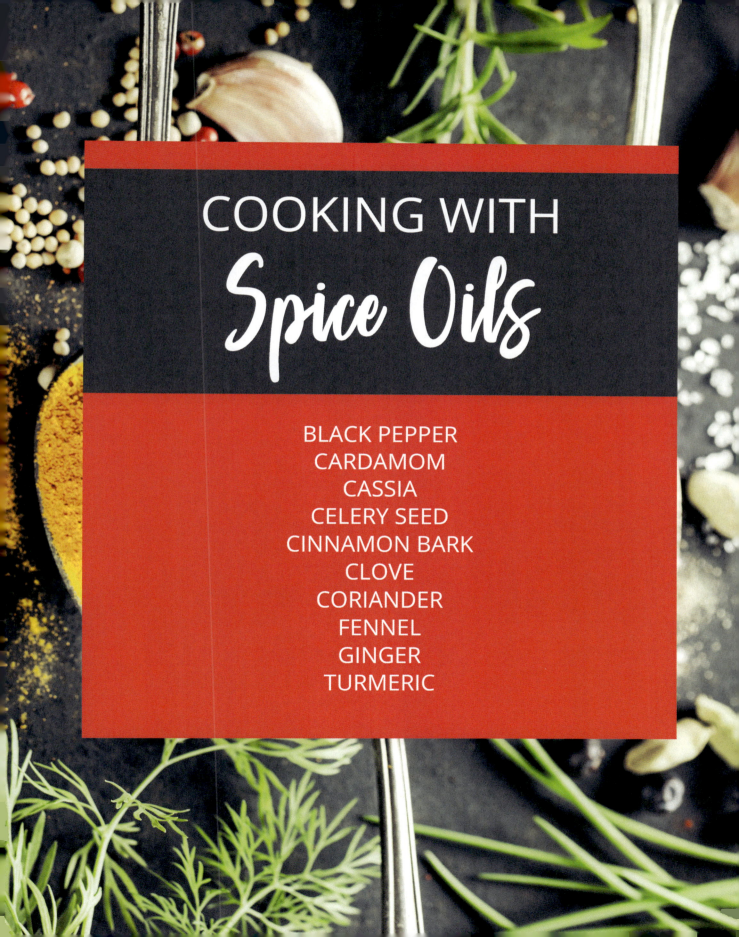

Top Uses of Spice Oils

The spice oils have a warming property, making them ideal for aiding in digestive issues and immune support. They add a warm, spiced, and cozy feeling to any dish, taking your meals to the next level.

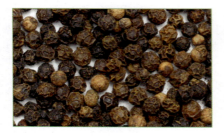

Black pepper

Constipation, diarrhea and gas, respiratory and lymphatic drainage and cleansing, poor circulation and cold extremities, cold, flu, aches and chills, congested airways, anxiety, cramps, sprains and muscle spasms, smoking, emotional balance

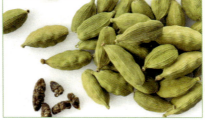

Cardamom

Congestion, stomachache and constipation, colitis and diarrhea, gastritis and stomach ulcers, menstrual and muscular pain, sore throat and fever, mental fatigue and confusion, pancreatitis, bad breath and household odors, emotional balance

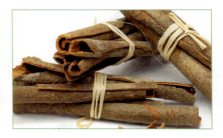

Cassia

Cold extremities, upset stomach and vomiting, detox for ear, nose, throat and lungs, water retention and kidney infection, viruses and bacteria, blood sugar balance, metabolism boost, sexual drive, emotional balance

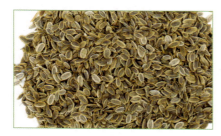

Celery Seed

Celery juice alternative, edema, urinary health, blood and liver toxicity, detox, weak and stiff joints, gout, arthritis and rheumatism, osteoporosis, high blood pressure and restricted blood flow, indigestion, flatulence, diarrhea, poor appetite, peripheral nerve damage and neuropathy, weakened spinal discs, kidney, bladder or gallstones, ulcers, gerd and stomach lining issues, headache and dizziness, epilepsy and stroke, irregular menstrual flow and cramps, uterine health, insect repellent, emotional balance

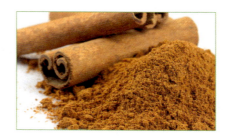

Cinnamon bark

Diabetes and high blood sugar, cold and flu, cholesterol and heart issues, oral health, fungus and bacteria, kidney infection, vaginal health, low libido and sexual stimulant, muscle strain and pain, emotional balance

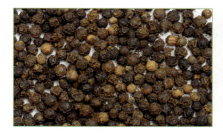

Clove

Liver and brain support, immune boost, circulation and hypertension, tooth pain and cavities, thyroid issues and metabolism support, infection and parasites, smoking addiction, virus and cold, emotional balance

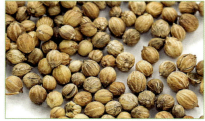

Coriander

Gas and nausea, high blood sugar and diabetes, itchy skin and rashes, joint pain, neuropathy, no appetite, food poisoning and diarrhea, body odor, low energy and nervous exhaustion, emotional balance

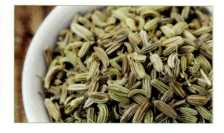

Fennel

Nausea, colic and flatulence, menstrual issues and PMS, menopause and premenopause issues, cramps and spasms, breast-feeding or low milk supply, edema and fluid retention, cough and congestion, intestinal parasites and sluggish bowels, blood sugar imbalance and hunger pains, stroke, emotional balance

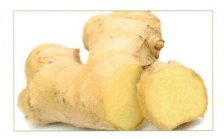

Ginger

Spasms, cramps and sore muscles, nausea, morning sickness and loss of appetite, motion sickness and vertigo, memory and brain support, heartburn and reflux, alcohol addiction, hormone and blood sugar imbalances, colic and constipation, neurotransmitter deficiencies, congestion, sinusitis and laryngitis, cold, flu, sore throat, sprains, broken bones, emotional balance

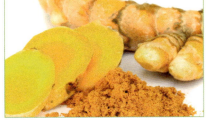

Turmeric

Cancer and tumors, autoimmune disorders, joint pain and swelling, arthritis, gout, rheumatism, fungal, bacterial, or viral infections, Alzheimer's, stroke, poor blood supply, blood and lymph purifier, liver and gallbladder detox, intestinal worms and parasites, acne, eczema and psoriasis, depression and discouragement, tension and anxiety, ulcers, gas and bloating, indigestion, compromised intestinal flora, poor circulation, diabetes and metabolism, high cholesterol, cough, respiratory issues and bronchitis, sore muscles and menstrual cramps, cavities and oral health, insect repellent, bites and stings, emotional balance

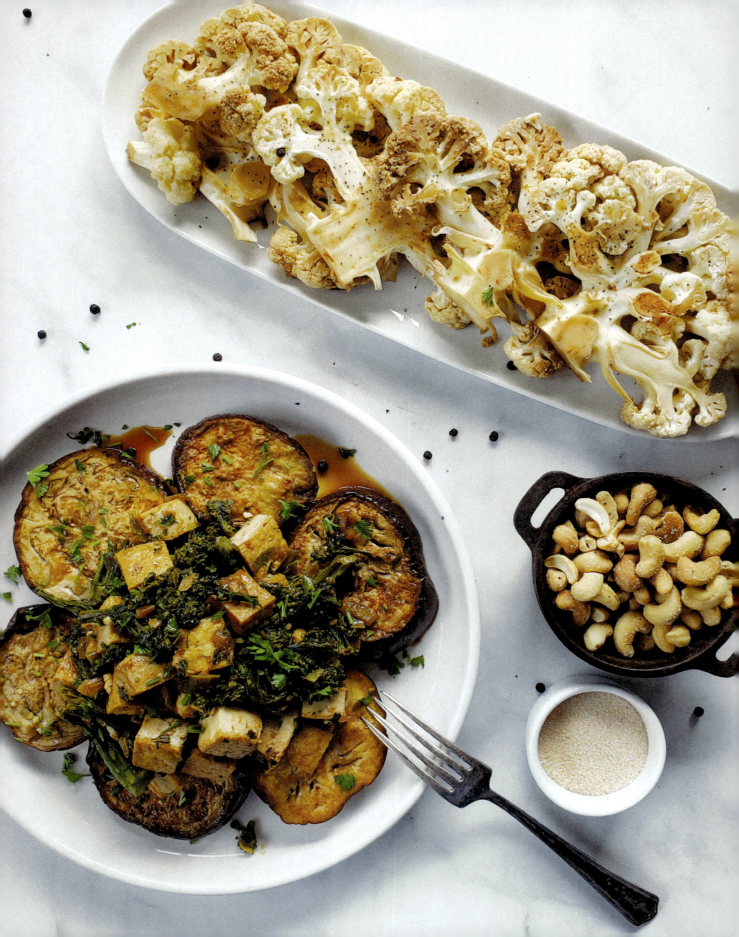

AROMA: *SPICY + SHARP* | **FLAVORS:** *PUNGENT*
PAIRS WITH: *VEGETABLES* | **MAIN USES:** *CIRCULATION*

Black Pepper

MARINATED CAULIFLOWER STEAK

2 cauliflower steaks
1/4 cup rice vinegar
1 T tamari, low sodium
1/2 t liquid smoke
2 drops Black Pepper essential oil

Combine liquids in glass container before adding cauliflower steaks to marinate for 3-4 hours. Roast at 400°F until golden and tender, about 20-30 minutes.

SIMPLE SEASONING SALT

3 T Himalayan pink salt
3 drops Black Pepper essential oil
1 T granulated garlic

Combine in small bowl and sprinkle over your dishes to taste—a pinch to a 1/4 tsp per plate is a good start.

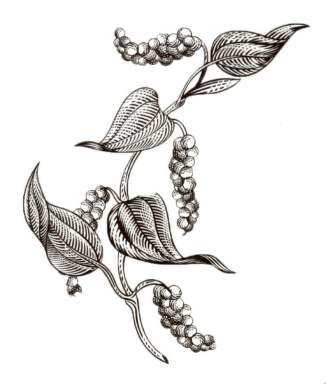

BLACK PEPPER ROASTED CASHEWS

2 cups cashews
1/4 t avocado oil
1/4 t salt
2 drops Black Pepper essential oil

1. Roast nuts plain at 250°F for 15-17 minutes.
2. Combine oils in bowl before adding nuts.
3. Season with salt to taste. Return to oven for 3 more minutes to set seasoning.

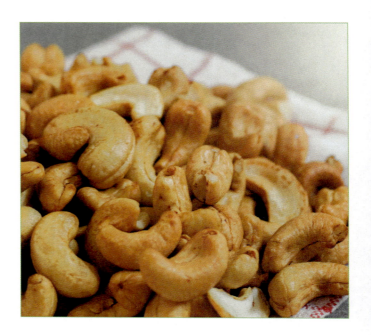

Try this! Marinate tofu, tempeh, or mushrooms in steak seasoning.

EGGPLANT STEAK

1 eggplant, cut into 1" thick steaks
1/4 cup rice vinegar
1 T tamari, low sodium
1/2 t liquid smoke
1 t maple syrup
2 drops Black Pepper essential oil
1/2 t garlic powder
1/2 t onion powder
1/4 t ground mustard
1/4 t smoked paprika

Combine liquids and spices in glass container before adding eggplant steaks to marinate for 3-4 hours. Roast at 400°F until golden and tender, about 15-20 minutes.

CRISPY BLACK PEPPER TOFU

1/2 cup low sodium tamari
3 T maple syrup
3 T rice vinegar
2 cloves garlic, pressed

1 drop Ginger essential oil
1 drop Black Pepper essential oil

1 package extra firm tofu, drained, pressed, and cut into cubes
1 bunch scallions, whites for sauteing and greens for garnishing
1/2 pound broccolini

1. Combine tamari, maple syrup, vinegar, and garlic in a sauce pot and reduce over medium heat, about 15 minutes.
2. Add essential oils when the sauce is thick and remove from heat and set aside.
3. Pan "fry" the tofu in a skillet lined with parchment paper. Remove from the pan and set aside when finished.
4. In the same skillet, saute the chopped scallion whites for a few minutes. Add chopped broccolini and cook on medium/high heat until bright green, about 4 minutes.
5. Add the tofu and the sauce to the skillet, stirring to coat. Garnish with the sliced scallion greens and sesame seeds. Serve with rice or quinoa.

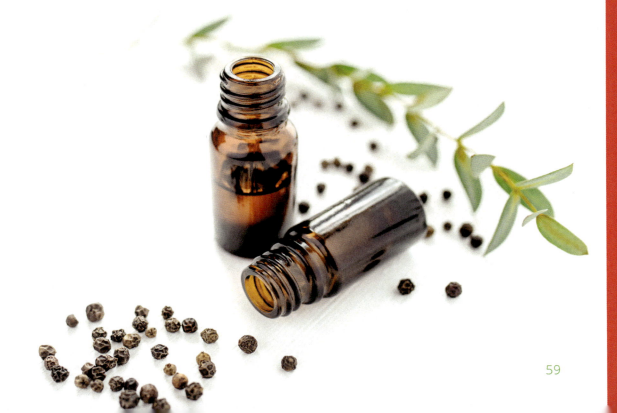

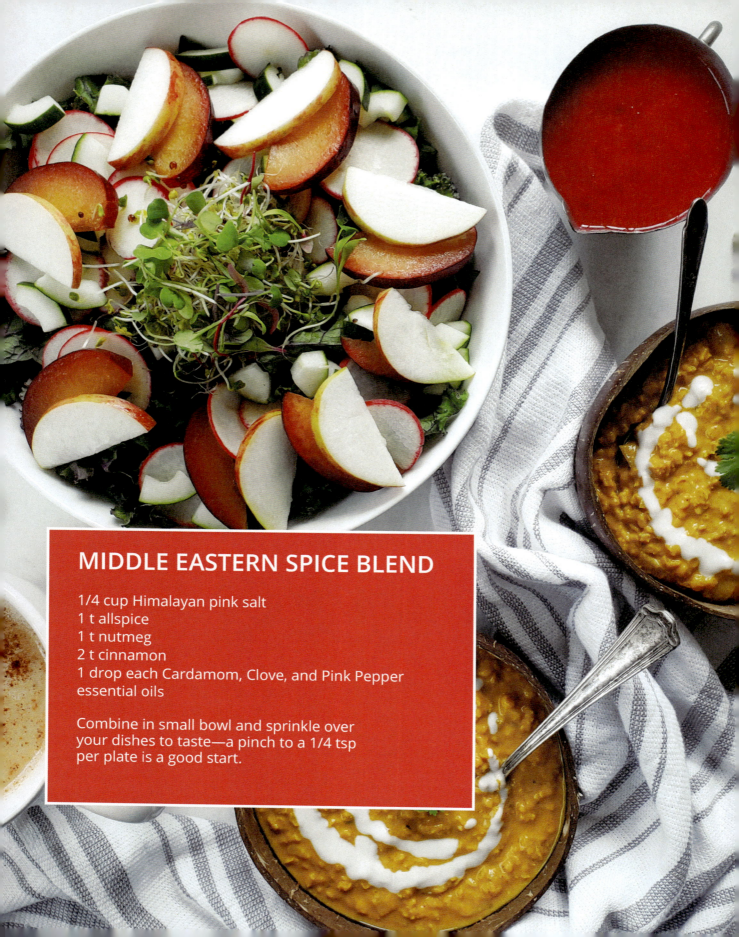

MIDDLE EASTERN SPICE BLEND

1/4 cup Himalayan pink salt
1 t allspice
1 t nutmeg
2 t cinnamon
1 drop each Cardamom, Clove, and Pink Pepper essential oils

Combine in small bowl and sprinkle over your dishes to taste—a pinch to a 1/4 tsp per plate is a good start.

AROMA: SPICY + WARM | FLAVORS: CITRUS + SPICE
PAIRS WITH: GINGER + SQUASH | MAIN USES: RESPIRATORY

Cardamom

APPLE, RADISH, AND PLUM SALAD

Salad:
1 medium apple, cut into matchsticks
1 red plum, cut into wedges
2 medium watermelon radishes, cut into matchsticks
1 cucumber, seeded and diced
2 cups kale, stemmed and shredded

Dressing:
3 red plums, cut into wedges
1 t coconut sugar or maple syrup
1/2 t salt
1/4 cup orange juice
2 T apple cider vinegar
1/4 t crushed red pepper

2 t lime juice
1 drop each Ginger and Cardamom essential oils

1. Add salad ingredients to a medium bowl.
2. In a sauce pot, heat the plum with the sugar and salt until the juices release and reduce. Add all other dressing ingredients and simmer for 10 minutes.
3. Remove from heat and finish with lime juice and essential oils. Puree with immersion blender if needed before dressing the salad.

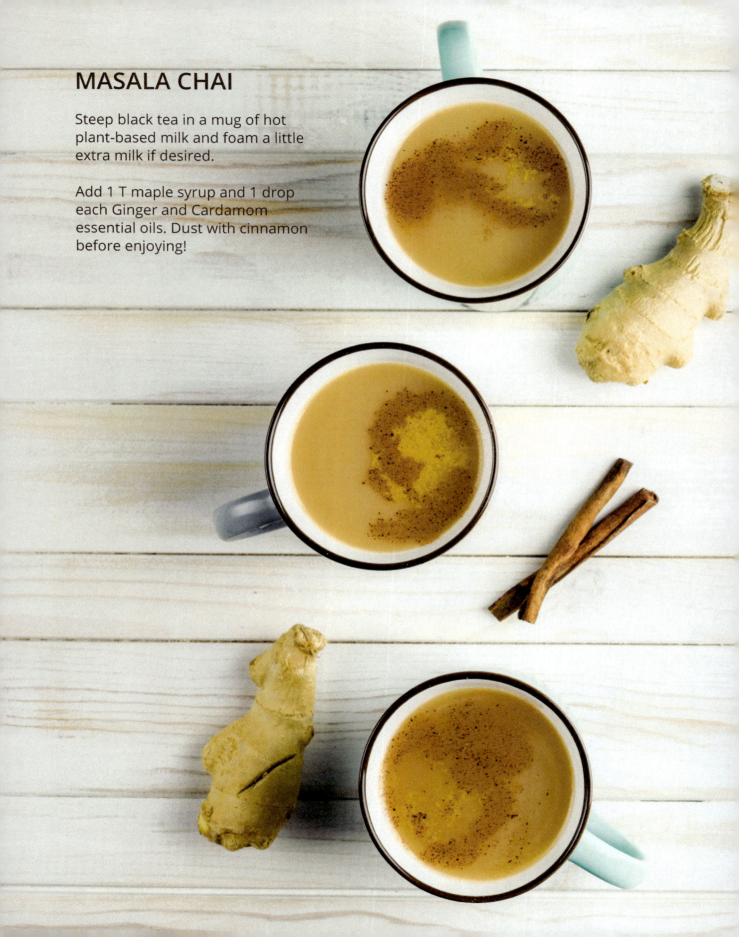

MASALA CHAI

Steep black tea in a mug of hot plant-based milk and foam a little extra milk if desired.

Add 1 T maple syrup and 1 drop each Ginger and Cardamom essential oils. Dust with cinnamon before enjoying!

LENTIL TIKKA MASALA

1 yellow onion, diced
2 cloves garlic, freshly grated

1 t Himalayan pink salt
1/2 t black pepper
1 t paprika
1 T curry powder
1/2 t cayenne
1/2 t cinnamon
1 t cumin
1 t turmeric
1 can tomato paste

2 cups red lentils
4 cups vegetable broth, low sodium
1 bay leaf

1 can coconut milk
1 drop Ginger essential oil
1 drop Cardamom essential oil

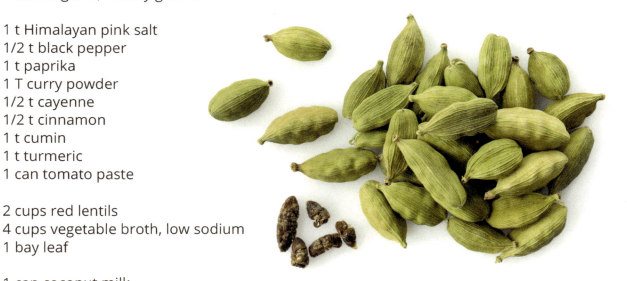

1. Cook onion on medium heat in a soup pot until fragrant and soft, about 4 minutes. Add the garlic and cook one minute more.
2. Add the spices and tomato paste. Stir for 1-2 minutes to warm spices.
3. Add the lentils, broth, and bay leaf and bring to a low boil. Reduce heat to simmer, covered, for about 20 minutes. The lentils should be slightly underdone.
4. Add the coconut milk and essential oils and cook for 5-10 minutes more, until lentils are tender.

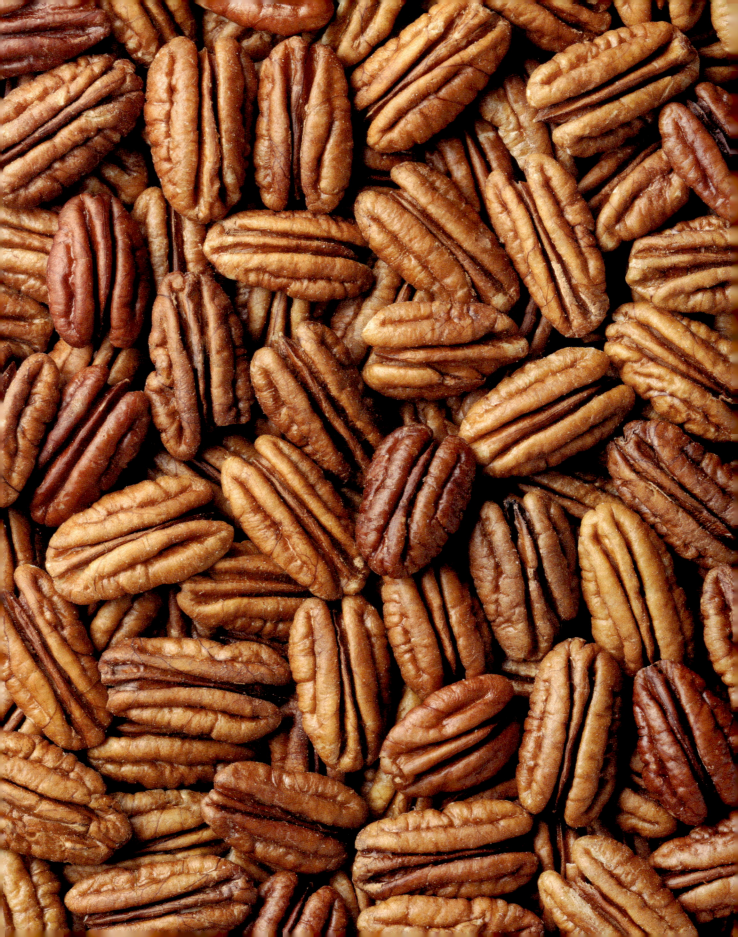

AROMA: *SPICY + CINNAMON* | **FLAVORS:** *SWEET + STRONG*
PAIRS WITH: *LENTILS + ROOTS* | **MAIN USES:** *DIGESTION*

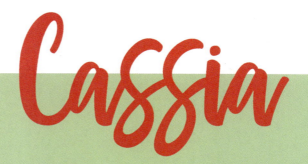

Cassia

CASSIA ROASTED PECANS

2 cups pecans
1/4 t avocado oil
2 drops Cassia essential oil

1. Roast nuts plain at 250°F for 12-15 minutes.
2. Combine oils in bowl before adding nuts.
3. Season with salt, coconut sugar, and cinnamon to taste.

PUMPKIN SPICE POPCORN

1. Pop organic popcorn kernels in an air popper.
2. In a small bowl, add 3 T melted coconut oil and 1 drop each Cassia and Clove essential oils.
3. Toss with popcorn and sprinkle with Himalayan pink salt, coconut sugar, and cinnamon.

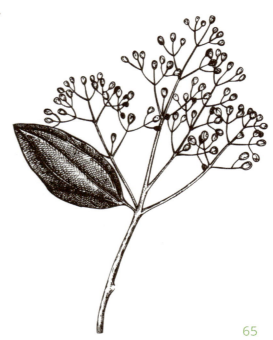

CINNAMON CHOCOLATE TRUFFLES

1 can coconut milk, refrigerated overnight—use top cream only
1 bag dairy free chocolate chips, such as Enjoy Life mini chocolate chips
1 drop Cassia essential oil

Melt coconut cream and chocolate chips until smooth. Stir in essential oil and refrigerate until firm but still soft enough to scoop into truffles. Roll in cacao powder, coconut flakes, or a mixture of both with a dash of ground cinnamon!

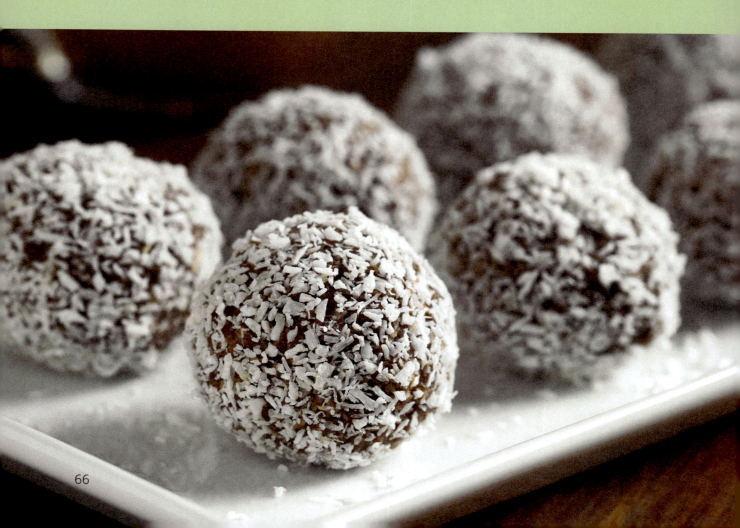

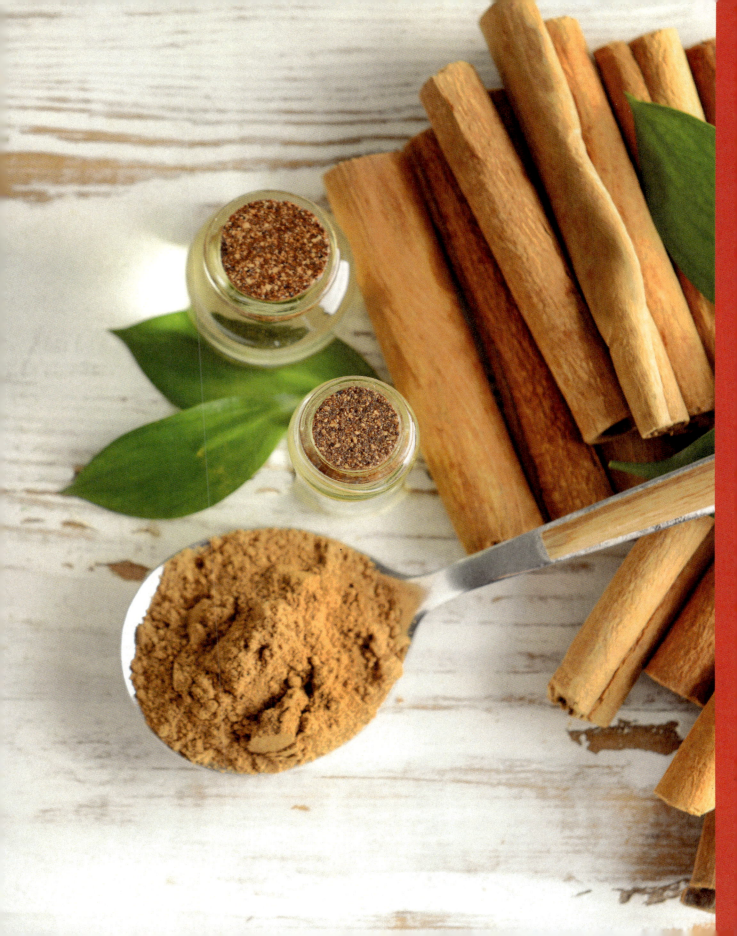

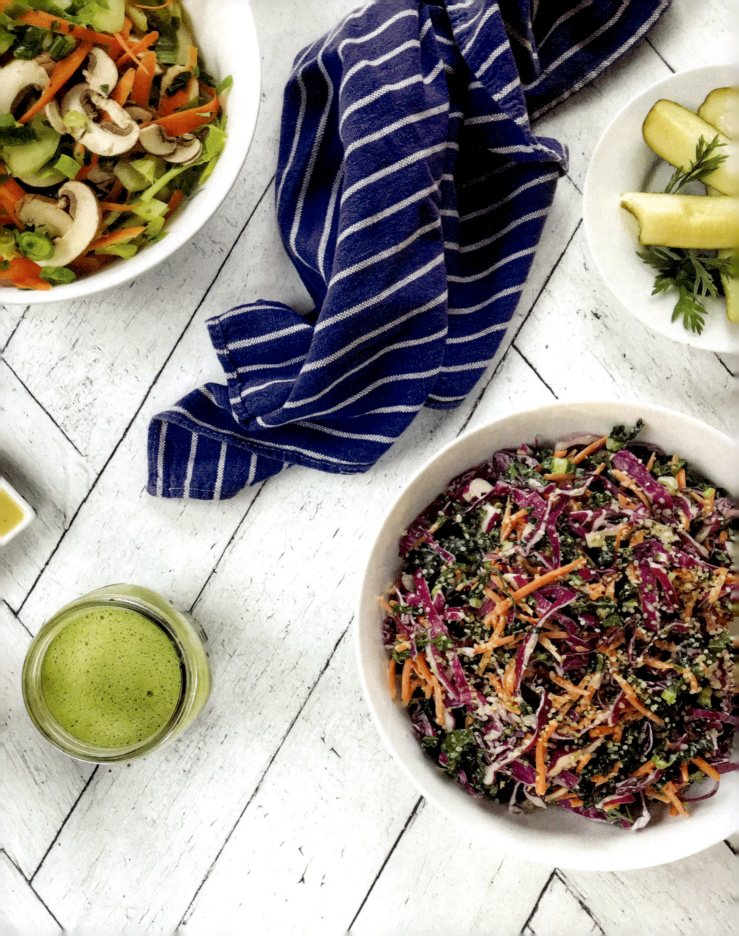

AROMA: *EARTHY + SPICY* | **FLAVORS:** *GRASSY + BITTER*
PAIRS WITH: *DILL + PICKLING* | **MAIN USES:** *URINARY + ELIMINATION*

Celery Seed

RAINBOW SLAW

Salad:
1 head kale, shredded
1 cup shredded carrots
1 cup shredded red cabbage
1 cup shredded brussels sprouts

Dressing:
1/4 cup vegan mayo
1/4 cup apple cider vinegar
2 T maple syrup
1/4 t salt
1/4 t pepper
1 drop Celery Seed essential oil

1. In a medium bowl, add the dressing ingredients and whisk until combined.
2. Add the salad ingredients and toss until well coated. Serve immediately.

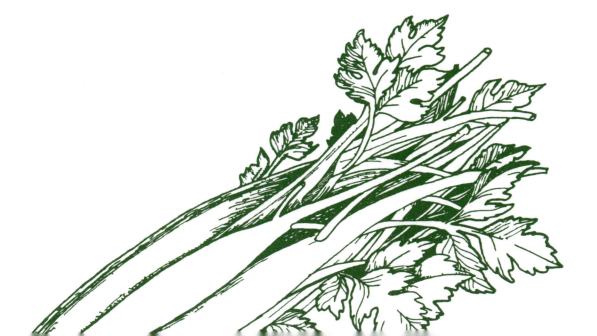

CELERY SALAD WITH VINAIGRETTE

Salad:
2 carrots, peeled into ribbons
3 celery stalks, sliced thinly on a bias
1 bunch parsley, chopped.
1 cup button mushrooms, sliced thin
1 bunch scallions, sliced thin

Dressing:
1/4 cup extra-virgin olive oil
1 clove garlic, pressed
2 T apple cider vinegar
1 T maple syrup
1 drop Celery seed essential oil
1/4 t salt
1/4 t ground mustard

1. Add all salad ingredients to a bowl.
2. Make the dressing in a blender, pour over salad before serving.

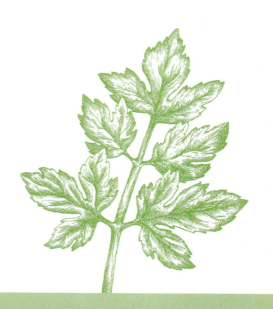

SUPER JUICE

4-6 kale stems
1-2 cucumber
4-6 stalks fresh celery
1/2 green apple
1 drop Celery Seed essential oil

Juice all produce, adding essential oil before enjoying.

QUICK PICKLES

6 cucumbers, sliced into spears
2 T rice vinegar or apple cider vinegar
1/2 t maple syrup
Pinch red pepper flakes
1 t Himalayan pink salt

1 T fresh dill, chopped
1 T lemon juice
1 drop Celery Seed essential oil

1. Toss cucumbers and spices in a bowl and chill for 1-6 hours.
2. Combine dill, lemon, and essential oil in a small dish before adding to the bowl to disperse the essential oil.

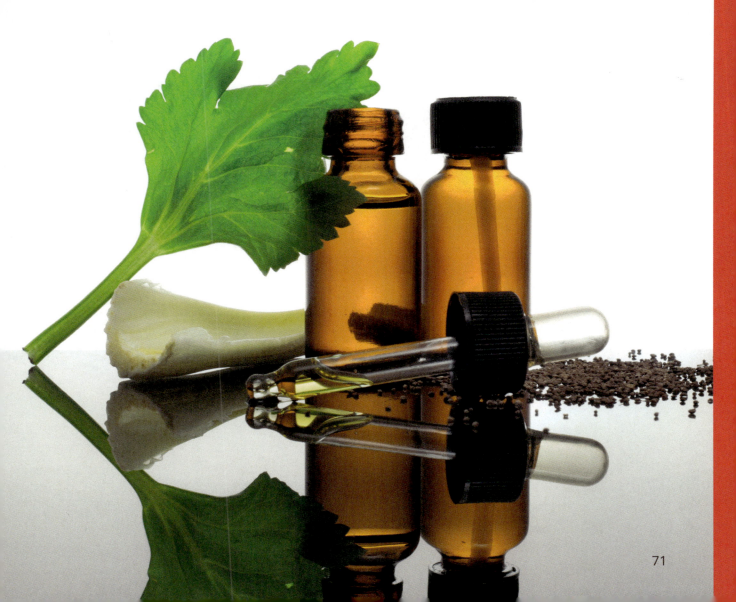

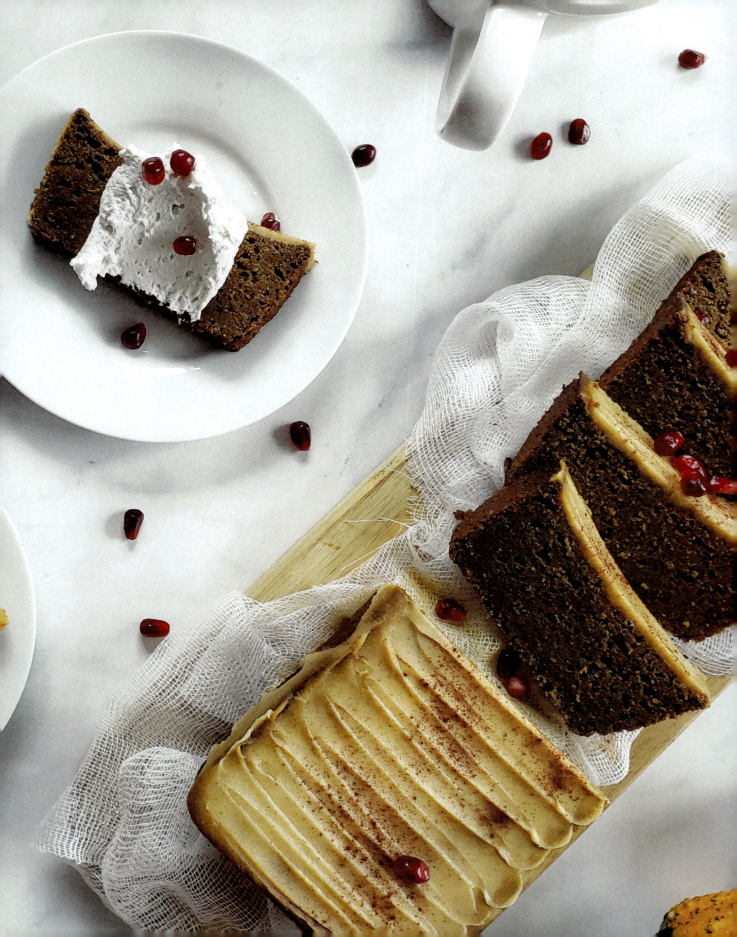

AROMA: *WOODY + SWEET* | **FLAVORS:** *SWEET + SPICY*
PAIRS WITH: *SQUASH + CACAO* | **MAIN USES:** *METABOLISM*

Cinnamon Bark

HOLIDAY GLAZED GINGERBREAD

3/4 cup chickpea flour
3/4 cup brown rice flour
1/2 cup potato starch
3/4 t xanthan gum
1/2 t nutmeg
1/2 t salt
1 t baking powder
1/2 t baking soda

1/2 cup melted coconut oil
1/3 cup blackstrap molasses
1 t vanilla
2 T apple cider vinegar
1 1/4 cup almond milk
1/2 cup applesauce
2/3 cup coconut sugar
4 drops Ginger essential oil
2 drops Cinnamon Bark essential oil

1. Add dry ingredients to bowl and whisk to combine.
2. Combine wet ingredients and whisk well in separate bowl before adding to dry ingredients.
3. Pour batter into greased loaf pan and bake at 325°F for 40-45 minutes.
4. To glaze, mix 1/4 cup melted coconut butter with 2 T maple syrup, 1/4 t cinnamon and 1 toothpick cinnamon bark. Add hot water 1 T at a time until thin enough to pour and spread on cooled loaf.

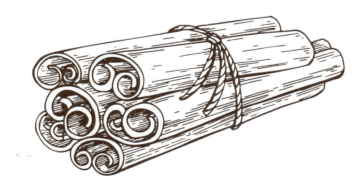

SWEET POTATO WAFFLES

1/4 cup flaxmeal
1/2 cup water

4 cups almond milk
1 t vanilla
2 t apple cider vinegar
3/4 cup sweet potato puree

3 cups gluten-free flour
1 cup oats
1/2 cup coconut sugar
1 t salt
2 t baking powder
1 t baking soda
1 t cinnamon
1 drop Cinnamon Bark essential oil

MAKES 10

1. Combine the flaxmeal with the water in a small bowl and let sit for 5-10 minutes.
2. Combine almond milk, vanilla, apple cider vinegar, and sweet potato puree in a bowl, whisking until smooth. Can substitute the sweet potato with canned pumpkin or butternut squash puree.
3. Combine all dry ingredients in a large bowl. Whisk in the sweet potato mixture and essential oil.
4. Let batter sit for 10 minutes before turning on your waffle iron.
5. Spray the waffle iron with coconut oil spray before each waffle is made.
6. Serve with mixed berries, spiced coconut cream, and maple syrup.

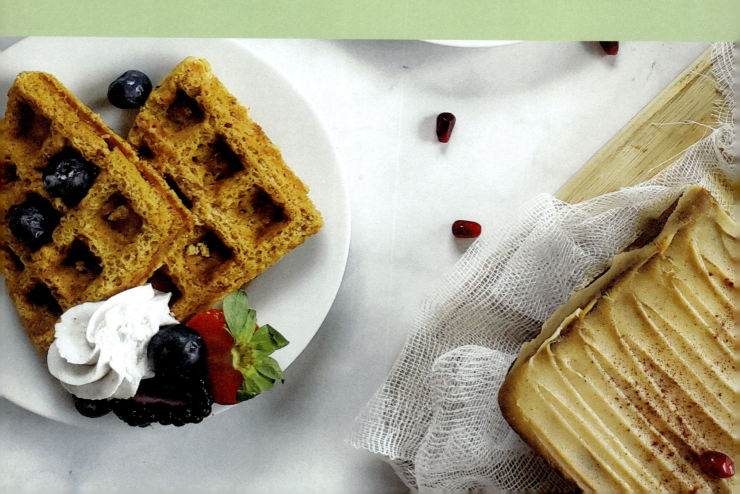

SPICED COCONUT CREAM

2 cans coconut milk, refrigerated overnight
2 T maple syrup
1 drop each Cinnamon Bark and Ginger essential oils
Dash nutmeg

1. Scoop top cream from cans into bowl and whip with a handheld beater fitted with the whisk attachment or in a stand mixer.
2. Add the maple syrup, essential oils, and nutmeg and mix until incorporated. Adjust sweetness and flavor as needed.

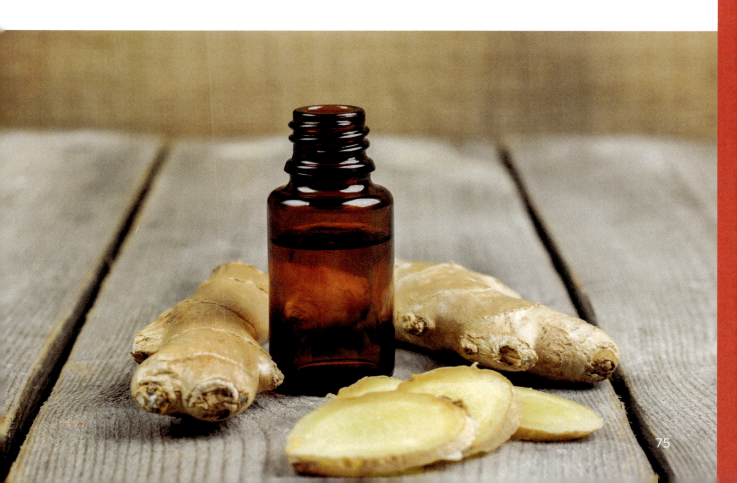

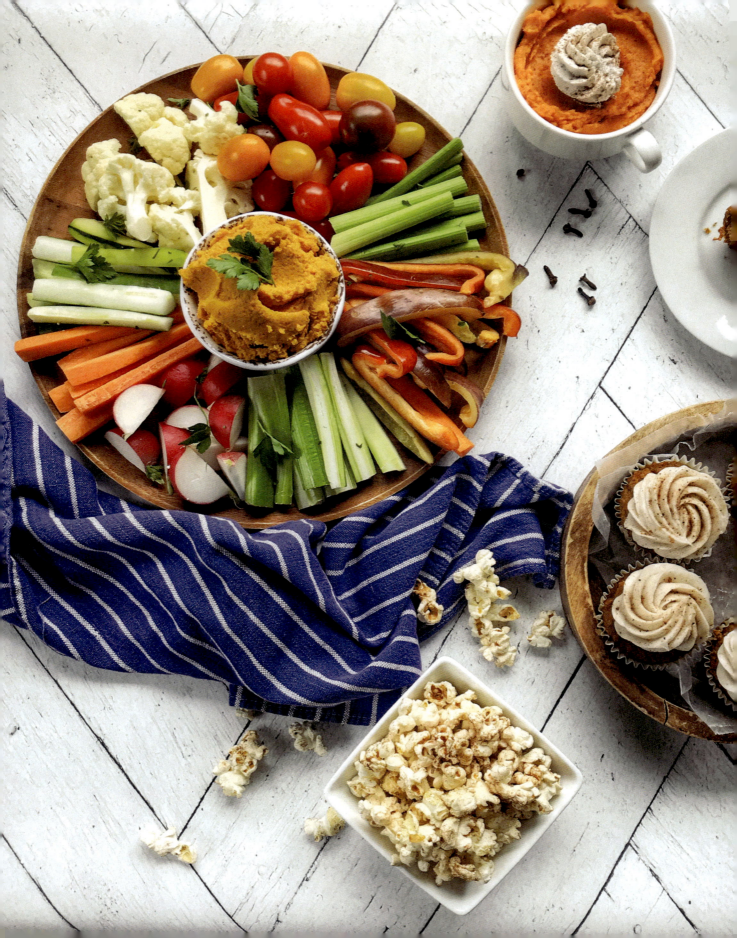

AROMA: WARM + WOODY | **FLAVORS:** STRONG + PUNGENT
PAIRS WITH: CITRUS | **MAIN USES:** ORAL CLEANSING

Clove

MOROCCAN CARROT HUMMUS

1 can chickpeas, drained and rinsed
2 cups cooked carrots, steamed or roasted
1 T tahini
1 clove garlic, freshly grated
1/2 t lemon juice
1/2 t cumin
1 drop each of Clove and Cassia essential oils

Blend all in a food processor, adding broth or olive oil to smooth hummus to desired texture.

APPLE PIE SPICED POPCORN

1. Pop organic popcorn kernels in an air popper
2. In a small bowl, add 3 T Extra virgin olive oil and 1 drop each Clove and Cassia essential oils.
3. Toss with popcorn and sprinkle with Himalayan pink salt, coconut sugar, cinnamon, and nutmeg.

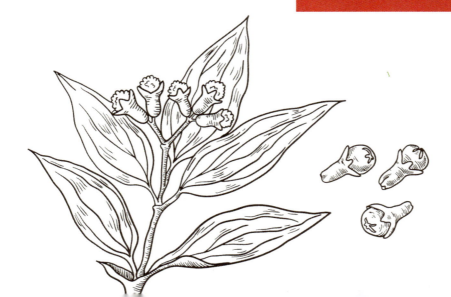

CHAI FROSTED SWEET POTATO CUPCAKES

3 T flax meal
1/2 cup water

1 cup sweet potato puree
1/4 cup maple syrup
1/3 cup melted coconut oil
2/3 cup coconut sugar
2/3 cup almond milk

1 1/2 cups GF flour
1 1/2 cups almond flour
1/2 T baking powder
1/2 T baking soda
1/4 t salt
1/2 T cinnamon

2 cups shredded carrots
4 drops Clove essential oil
2 drops Ginger essential oil

1. Combine flaxmeal and water in a large bowl to form flax egg, let sit 5 minutes.
2. Add all wet ingredients to the bowl with the flax egg.
3. Combine the dry ingredients in a separate bowl before sifting into the bowl of wet ingredients. Stir gently to combine.
4. Add essential oils and carrots and stir once more before portioning into sprayed or lined cupcake pans.
5. Bake at 375°F for 20 minutes and allow to cool for 5 minutes before removing from the pan.
6. Cool completely before frosting. Garnish with nutmeg, cinnamon, or chopped pecans.

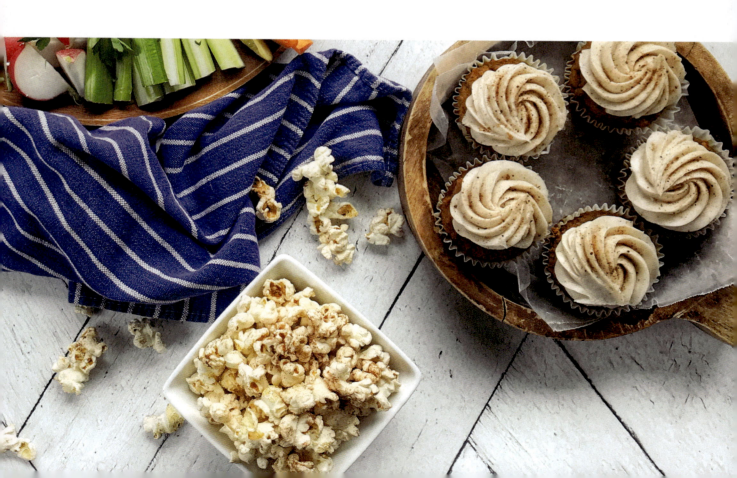

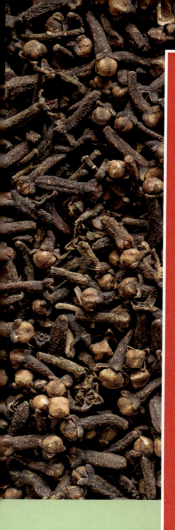
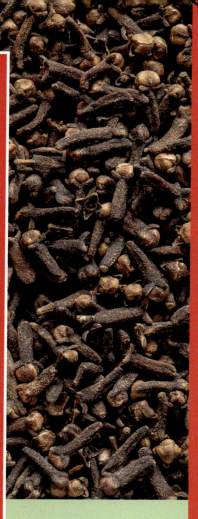

CHAI SPICED FROSTING

1 cup coconut oil, solidified but not cold

2 cans coconut milk

1/4 cup agave
1 t vanilla
1/4 cup melted coconut butter

1/4 t cinnamon
1 drop Clove essential oil
1 drop Cardamom essential oil
1 drop Ginger essential oil

1. Whip in bowl with paddle until smooth
2. Using the whisk attachment, add the top cream from canned coconut milk, agave, and vanilla and whip until fluffy
3. Add melted coconut butter in slowly while mixer is running. Whip until fluffy.
4. Drop in oils and cinnamon toward end of mixing. May need to switch back to paddle attachment.

SWEET POTATO PIE

Roast halved sweet potatoes face down on a sheet of parchment paper at 400°F until they're very soft, almost over baked, to bring out the natural sweetness. Remove skin once cooled and save for use in another recipe.

Whip sweet potato until fluffy and portion into bowls or glasses. Top with spiced coconut cream and a dash of nutmeg!

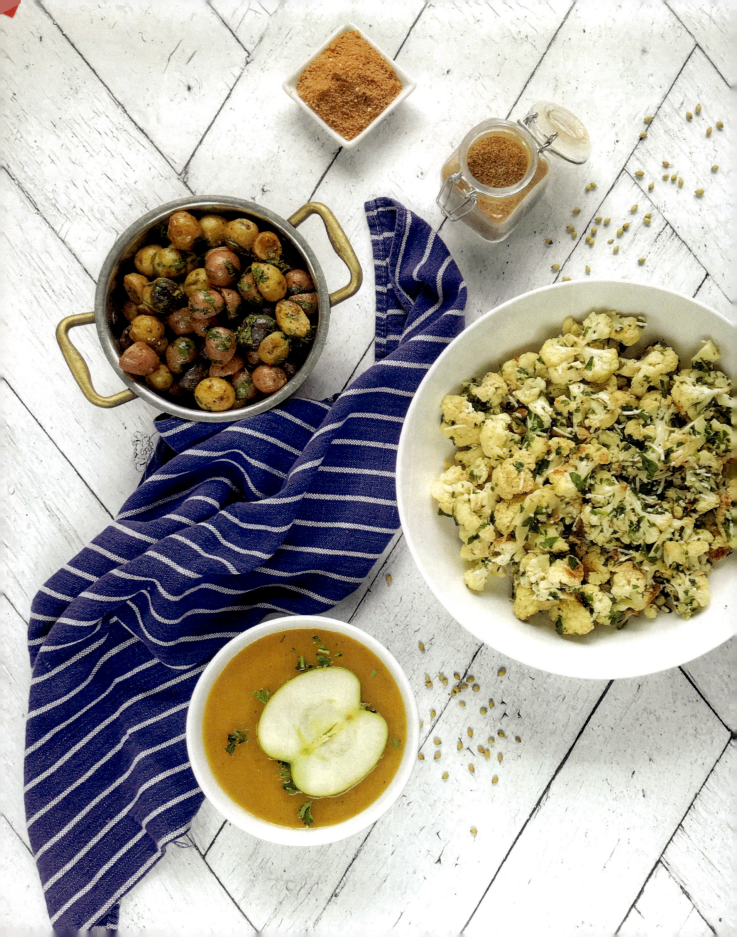

AROMA: *GREEN + SHARP* | **FLAVORS:** *WARM + NUTTY*
PAIRS WITH: *APPLES + CURRIES* | **MAIN USES:** *DIGESTION*

Coriander

SQUASH AND APPLE SOUP

1 medium onion, chopped
1 clove garlic, pressed

1 butternut squash, peeled and chopped
1 granny smith apple, peeled and chopped
1 golden delicious apple, peeled and chopped

4 cups vegetable broth
1 t salt
1/2 t nutmeg
1/4 t black pepper
1/4 t cayenne pepper

1 drop Coriander essential oil

Combining Golden Delicious and Granny Smith apples works really well!

1. Cook the onions in a soup pot over medium heat until fragrant and soft, about 4 minutes. Add the garlic and cook for one minute more.
2. Add the squash, apples, broth, and spices. Cook on medium/high heat until gently boiling.
3. Reduce heat to low, cover, and simmer until the vegetables are tender, about 20 minutes.
4. Remove from heat and puree with an immersion blender until smooth. Add more broth if a thinner soup is desired.
5. Add the essential oil to the pot before serving.

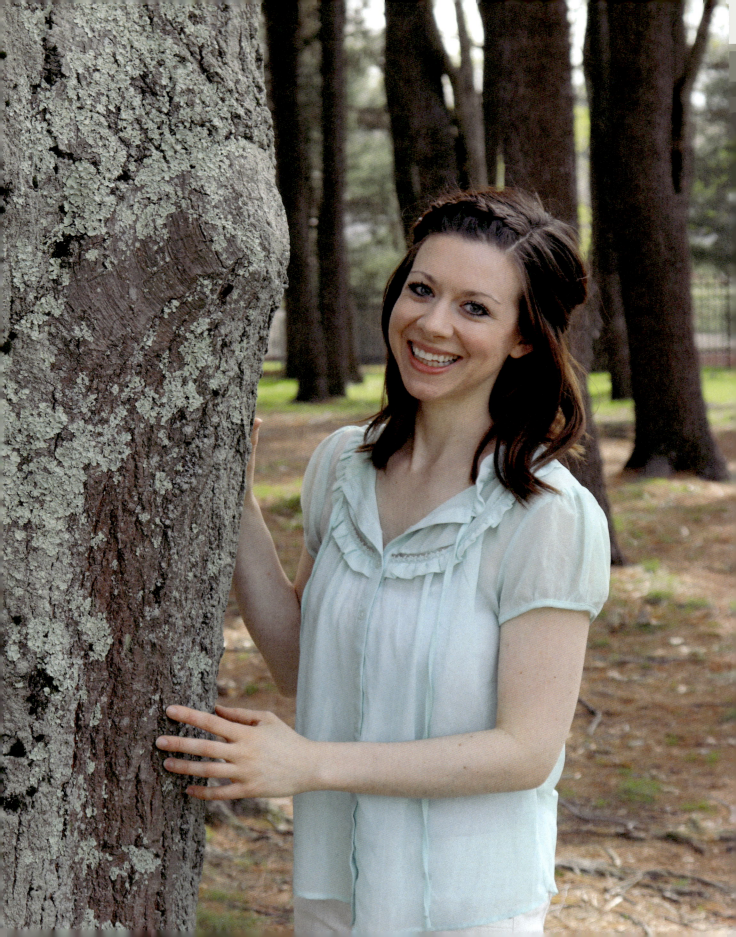

MOROCCAN SEASONING SALT

2 T paprika
1 T turmeric
2 1/2 t cinnamon
2 t ginger
1 1/2 t allspice
1 t black pepper
1 drop Cardamom essential oil
1 drop Coriander essential oil

Mix all spices in a small jar, add essential oils and stir to incorporate evenly.

Use on roasted vegetables, in hummus, or sprinkle over power bowls!

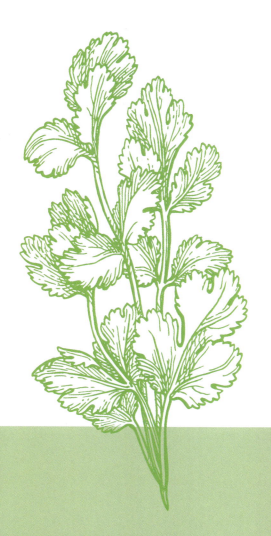

SPICED ROASTED POTATOES

2 T extra virgin olive oil
1 clove fresh pressed garlic
1/4 t salt
1/4 t black pepper
pinch cayenne pepper
1 drop Coriander essential oil

2-3 potatoes, your favorite type, chopped

1. Prepare the seasoning by combining all ingredients, except the potatoes, in a small bowl.
2. Roast the potatoes at 400°F for 15-20 minutes, or until cooked through.
3. Pour the seasoning mixture over the potatoes and stir until evenly coated.
4. Return the tray to the oven for 5 minutes to finish roasting.
5. Finish with a squeeze of fresh lemon juice and garnish with cilantro or add a few toothpicks of Cilantro essential oil to the seasoning mix!

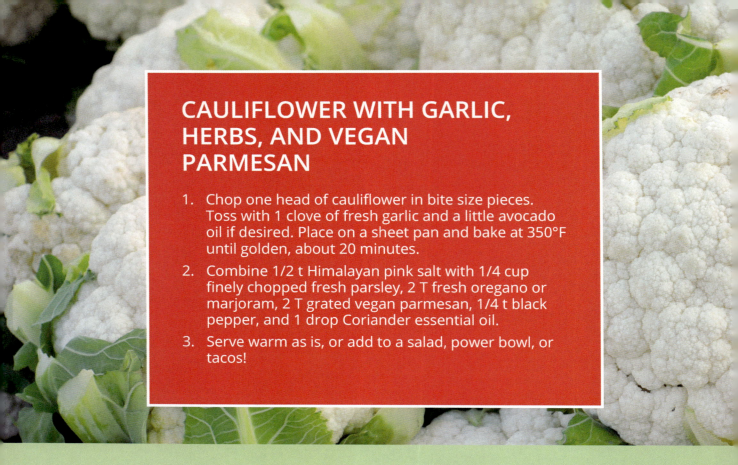

CAULIFLOWER WITH GARLIC, HERBS, AND VEGAN PARMESAN

1. Chop one head of cauliflower in bite size pieces. Toss with 1 clove of fresh garlic and a little avocado oil if desired. Place on a sheet pan and bake at 350°F until golden, about 20 minutes.

2. Combine 1/2 t Himalayan pink salt with 1/4 cup finely chopped fresh parsley, 2 T fresh oregano or marjoram, 2 T grated vegan parmesan, 1/4 t black pepper, and 1 drop Coriander essential oil.

3. Serve warm as is, or add to a salad, power bowl, or tacos!

SPICY CORIANDER SEASONING

1 t cumin
1 t white pepper
1 t cayenne pepper
2 t garlic powder
1 T Himalayan pink salt
1 drop Oregano essential oil
1 drop Thyme essential oil
3 drops Coriander essential oil

Mix all spices in a small jar, add essential oils and stir to incorporate evenly.

Use on portobello or cauliflower steaks, with jackfruit, or in marinades for your favorite root vegetables.

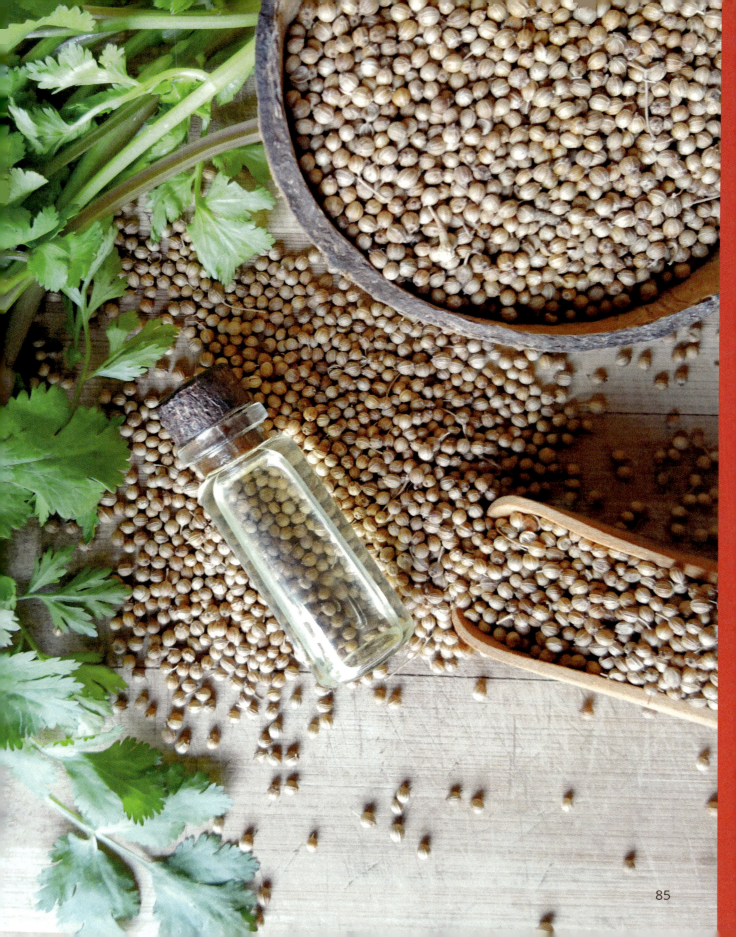

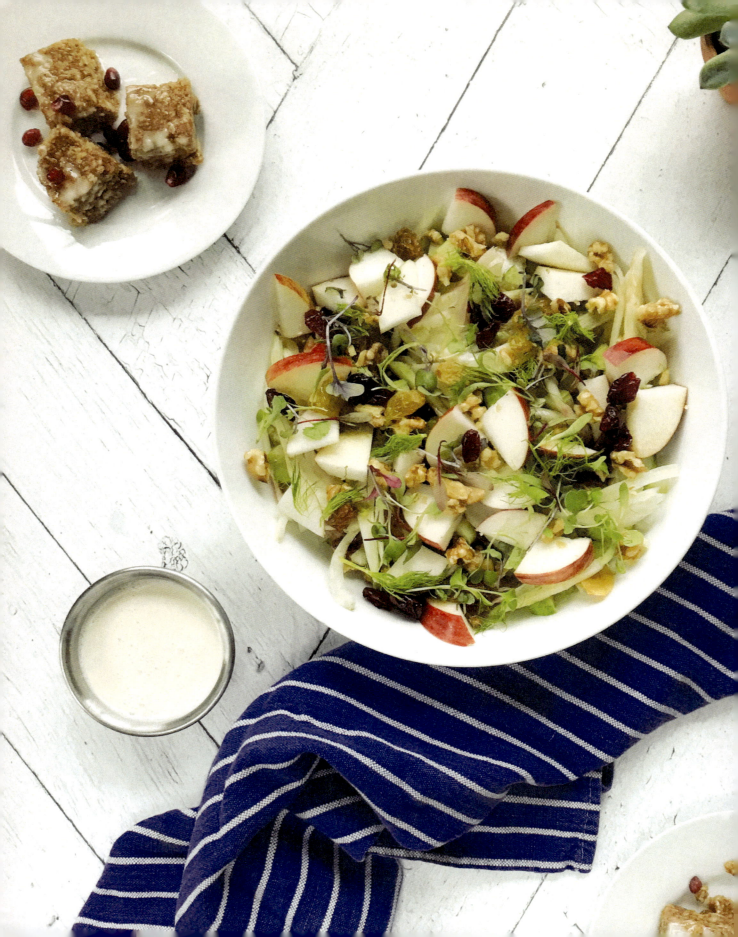

AROMA: LICORICE + HONEY | **FLAVORS:** SWEET + LICORICE
PAIRS WITH: CITRUS + HERBS | **MAIN USES:** DIGESTION

Fennel

CELERY AND APPLE SALAD WITH WALNUTS

1 head celery hearts, diced
1 fennel bulb, thinly sliced
3 cups your favorite greens
1 apple, diced and tossed in lemon juice
1/4 cup chopped walnuts
1/4 cup chopped dates or raisins

1. In a large bowl, make the dressing by whisking together 2 T apple cider vinegar, 2 T vegan mayo, 1 t maple syrup, and 1 drop of Fennel essential oil.
2. Add the salad ingredients and toss well before serving.

Essential oils are great to add to fresh juice for a burst of flavor and great internal benefits.

BRIGHT GREEN JUICE

Kale stems
3-4 celery stalks
1 cup spinach
2 apples
2 cucumbers

Juice all ingredients in a juicer and add one drop of Fennel essential oil.

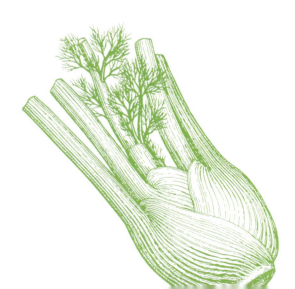

87

CHRISTMAS COOKIE OAT BITES

1 cup rolled oats
1 cup oat flour

1/2 cup almond milk
1 cup almond butter
1/4 cup melted coconut oil
1 t vanilla
1/4 cup maple syrup

1. In a medium bowl, combine the liquids, almond butter, and the Fennel essential oil.
2. Add the oats and oat flour, mix well.
3. Spread the mixture into a parchment lined loaf pan or 8x8 pan and place in the refrigerator to set for about 2 hours.
4. Mix a simple glaze by combining 1/4 cup melted coconut butter with 1/2 t vanilla, 1/4 t almond extract, and 1 drop Fennel essential oil. Add 1 T hot water at a time until just thin enough to spread—it will still be very thick though. Return to the refrigerator to set before slicing.

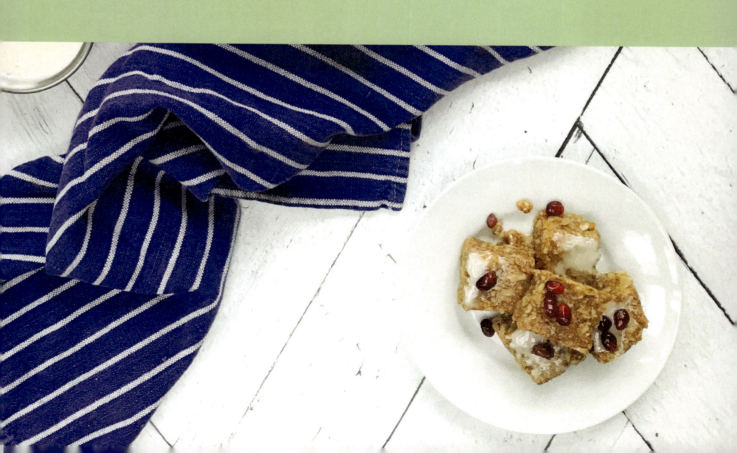

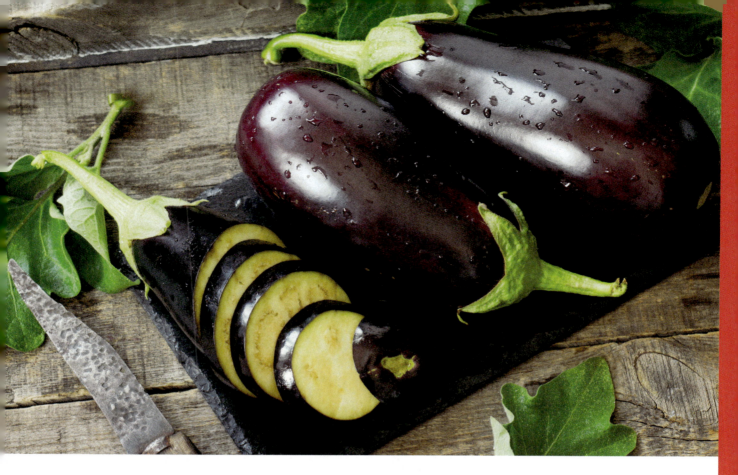

EGGPLANT PEPPERONI

1 t each salt and pepper
2 t crushed red pepper flakes
2 t ground mustard
2 t smoked paprika
2 t garlic powder
2 t coconut sugar
1/4 t ground anise
1 t liquid smoke
1 drop Fennel essential oil

1. Measure all ingredients into a glass or ceramic dish and mix until combined.
2. Slice one medium eggplant into 1/4-inch rounds and marinate for 4 hours or overnight for best flavor. Dehydrate at 135°F for 3-4 hours. If you don't have a dehydrator, bake the eggplant at your oven's lowest heat for 2-3 hours, checking on them regularly so they don't burn.
3. In both heating methods, make sure to rotate the eggplant for even dehydrating.
4. Enjoy on pizza, sandwiches, or as is!

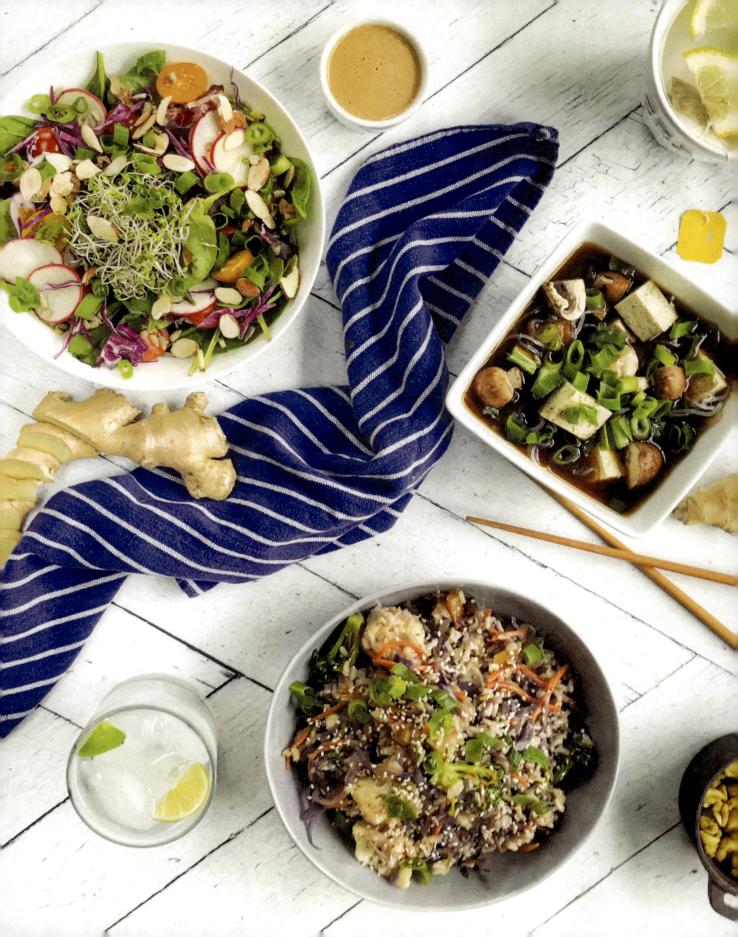

AROMA: SPICY + SWEET | **FLAVORS:** SPICY + WARM
PAIRS WITH: CITRUS + WARM SPICES | **MAIN USES:** DIGESTION

Ginger

ROASTED WASABI PEANUTS

2 cups unsalted peanuts

2 t wasabi powder
1/2 t salt
3 drops Ginger essential oil

1. Toss the peanuts in a little bit of melted coconut oil and roast at 300°F for 15 minutes.
2. Combine the wasabi powder, salt, and essential oil in a small dish before sprinkling over the roasted peanuts. Mix to distribute the seasoning evenly. Adjust seasoning as needed.
3. Enjoy in place of wasabi peas, add to a stir fry, or enjoy in a homemade savory trail mix!

ALMOND GINGER DRESSING

1/4 cup almond butter
1 t tamari
2 T rice vinegar
1/4 cup water
2 drops Ginger essential oil

Whisk in small bowl to combine and enjoy on salads, power bowls, or as a marinade.

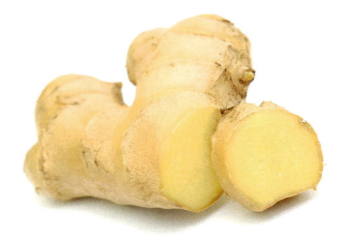

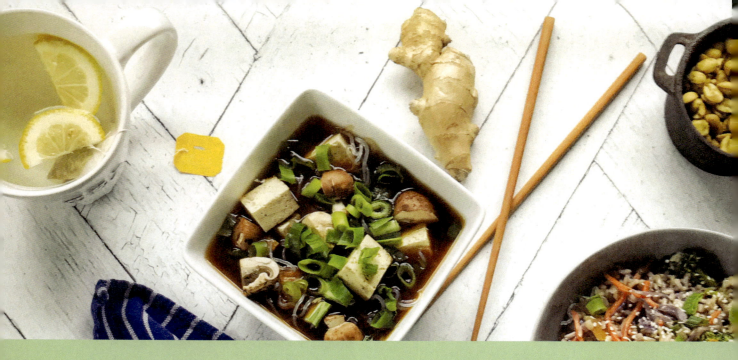

GINGER GARLIC STIR FRY SAUCE

1. Make stir fry as usual, using your favorite veggies and proteins.
2. In a small bowl, combine tamari and water in a 2:1 ratio.
3. Add fresh pressed garlic, 2 drops Ginger essential oil, and a little arrowroot, tapioca starch, or cornstarch to help thicken.
4. Continue cooking until sauce has thickened and coated veggies to your liking.
5. Make it as saucy as you like—I prefer to have extra so there is enough to cover the rice or quinoa too!

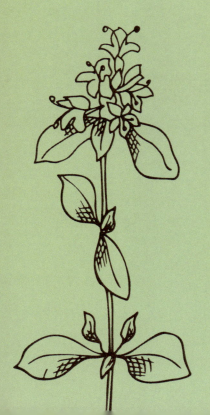

SORE THROAT SOOTHER TEA

1 1/2—2 cups water
1/3 cup apple cider vinegar
1/3 cup lemon juice
2 T raw honey
1-2 drops Ginger essential oil

Heat water on the kettle and place all remaining ingredients in a large mug. Pour in hot water and stir to melt honey before enjoying.

MISO BOWLS

2 T miso
1 T tamari
1 T rice vinegar
1/2 t toasted sesame oil

Assorted veggies:
-Asparagus or beans
-Greens
-Root veggies
-Mushrooms

1 clove garlic, freshly pressed
1 drop Ginger essential oil
Serves 3-4

FRESH GINGER BEER

1 drop Ginger essential oil
1/2 t maple syrup (optional)
8 oz sparkling water

Combine in glass and enjoy!

1. Combine in 4 cup measuring cup and set aside until ready to add hot water to create a broth to pour over the plated veggies.

2. Saute your assorted veggies, or heat up whatever you've got, until preferred texture is reached. I like my veggies to be a little crispy and crunchy for this dish.

3. *If using baked tofu or tempeh, add that here.

4. Add garlic and Ginger essential oil to broth along with enough hot water to equal 4 cups of finished broth before pouring over plated veggies. Top with sprouts or microgreens, scallions, or hemp seeds.

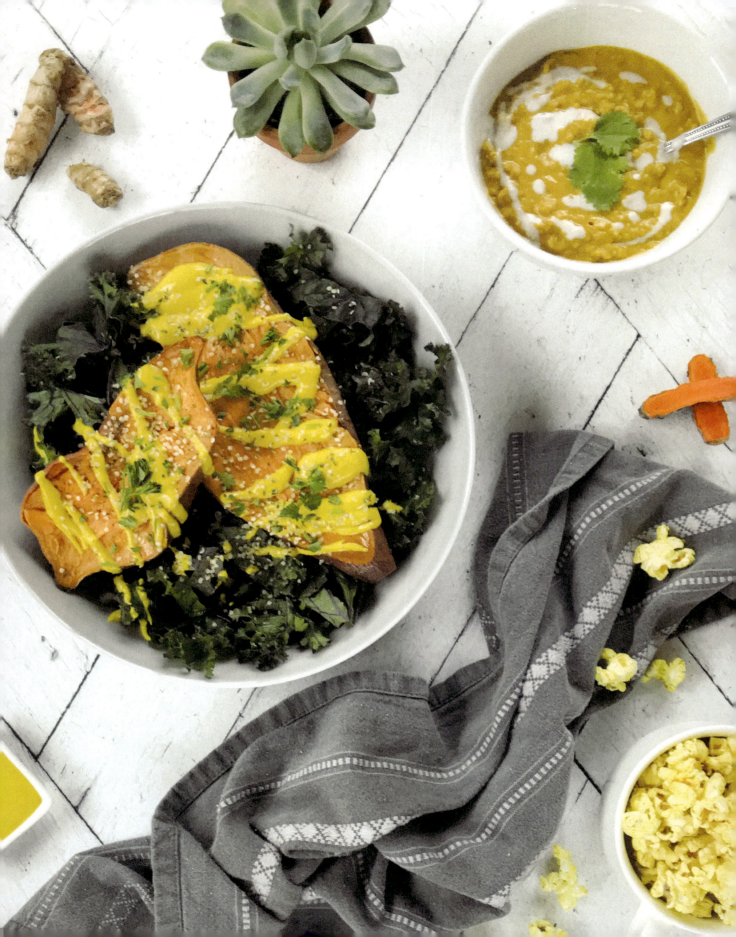

AROMA: *WOODY + EARTHY* | **FLAVORS:** *PUNGENT + BITTER*
PAIRS WITH: *CLOVE + GINGER* | **MAIN USES:** *NERVOUS + IMMUNE SYSTEMS*

Turmeric

TURMERIC DRESSING

1/4 cup tahini
1/4 cup apple cider vinegar
1 T maple syrup
1/4 t turmeric powder
1/4 t black pepper
1 drop Turmeric essential oil

Mix all ingredients with a whisk in a small bowl. Serve on anything!

GOLDEN MILK POPCORN

Organic popcorn
3 T extra-virgin olive oil
1 drop each Clove, Ginger, and Turmeric essential oils

1. Pop organic popcorn kernels in an air popper.
2. In a small bowl, mix extra-virgin olive oil and essential oils.
3. Toss the oils with the popcorn and sprinkle with Himalayan pink salt, coconut sugar, and cinnamon and turmeric powder.

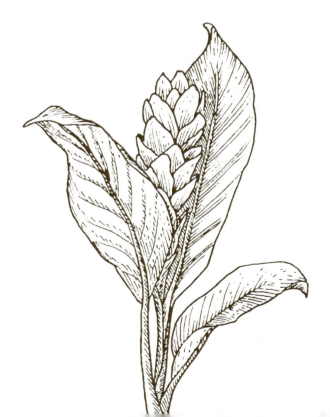

COCONUT RED LENTIL CURRY

1 yellow onion, diced
2 cloves garlic, freshly grated

1 t Himalayan pink salt
1/2 t black pepper
1 t paprika
1 T red curry paste
1/2 t cayenne
1/2 t cinnamon
1 t cumin
1 t turmeric
1 can tomato paste

2 cups red lentils
4 cups vegetable broth, low sodium
1 bay leaf
1 can coconut milk

1 drop Turmeric and Black Pepper essential oils

1. Cook the onion and garlic on medium heat in a soup pot until onion is soft and fragrant, about 4 minutes.
2. Add the spices and tomato paste and stir for 1-2 minutes.
3. Add lentils, broth and bay leaf and bring to boil. Reduce heat to simmer for about 20 minutes. Lentils should be slightly underdone.
4. Add coconut milk and essential oils and cook 5-10 minutes more, until lentils are fully tender.

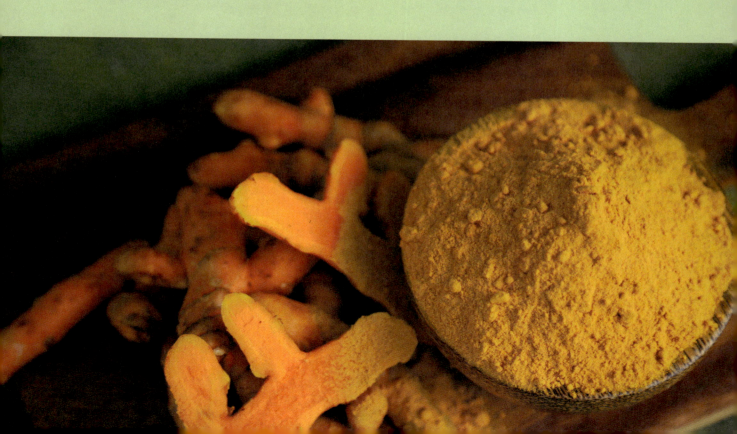

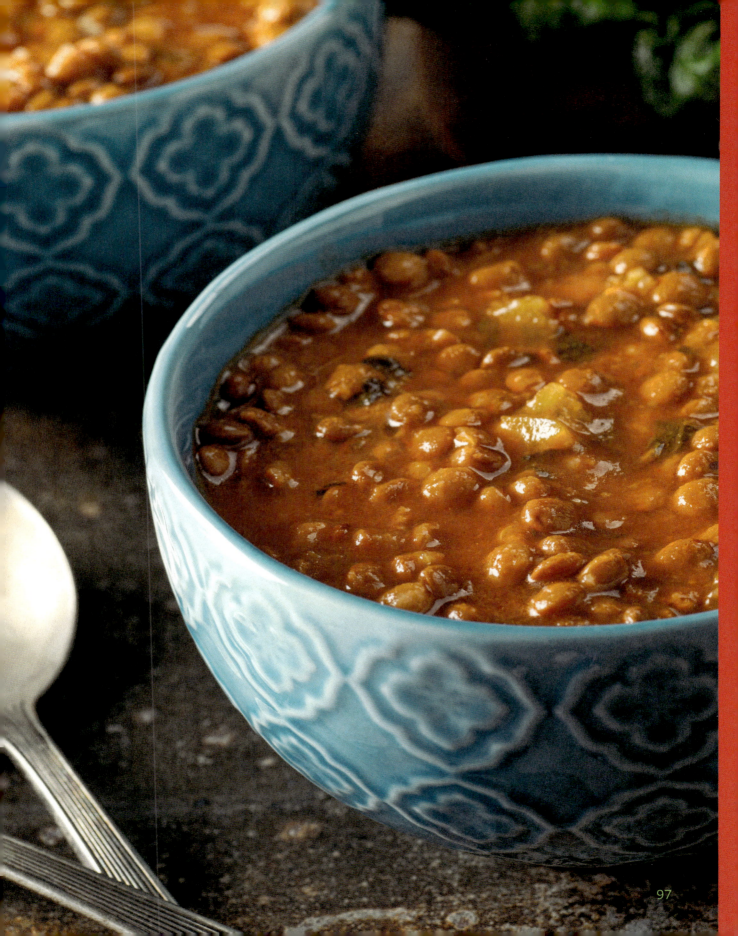

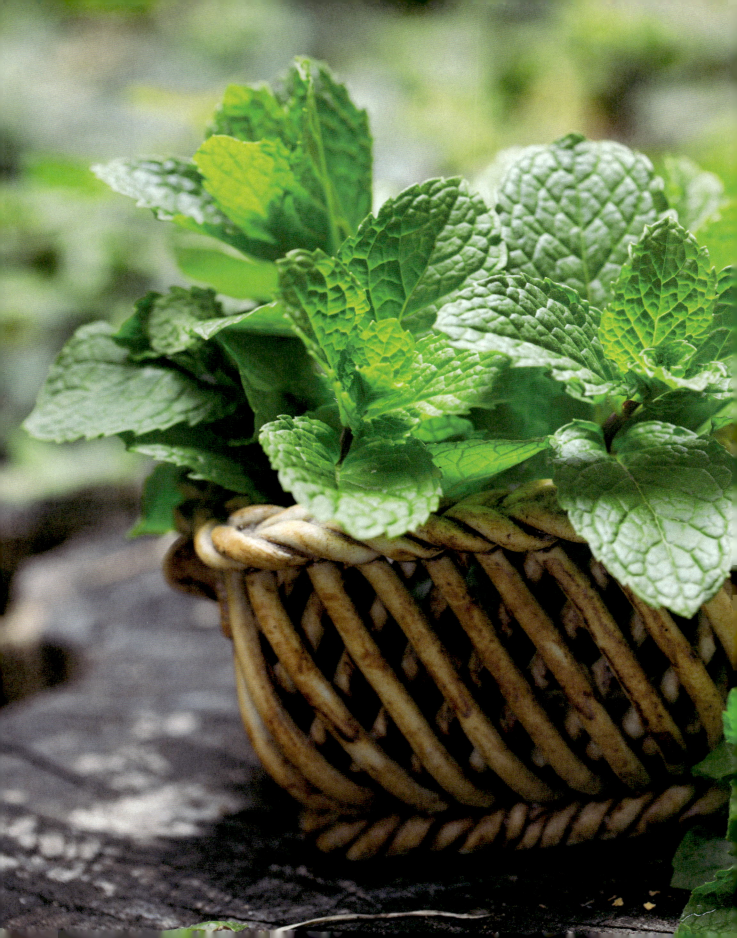

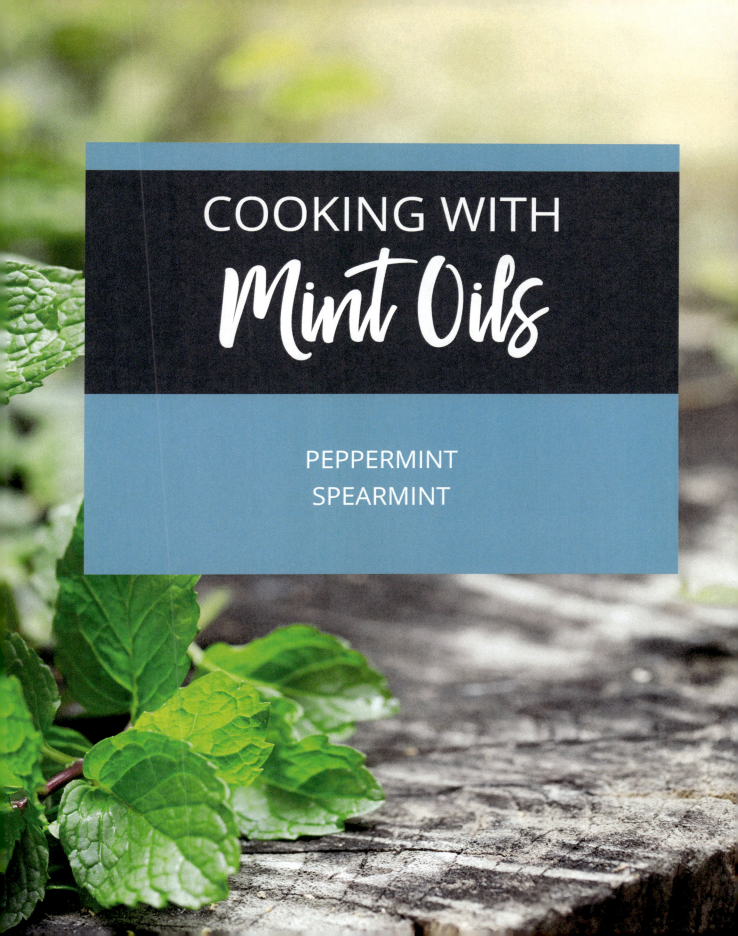

Top Uses for Mint Essential Oils

The mint oils are refreshing, relieving, and reenergizing. In addition to being a perfect freshener after a meal, mint oils can provide an interesting flavor to dressings, marinades, and desserts.

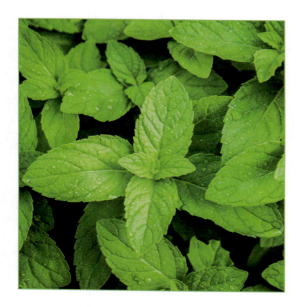

Peppermint

Alertness and energy, fevers and hot flashes, burns and sunburn, memory issues and autism, cravings, muscle stiffness and tension, allergies and hives, headaches and migraines, bad breath and hangover, asthma and sinusitis, decrease milk supply, loss of sense of smell, gastritis and digestive discomfort, gamma radiation exposure, emotional balance

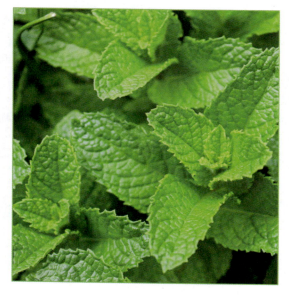

Spearmint

Indigestion, nausea and colic, bad breath, bronchitis and respiratory issues, acne, sores and scars, cooling, focus issues, depression and fatigue, stress and nervous issues, slow or heavy menstruation, headaches and migraines, emotional balance

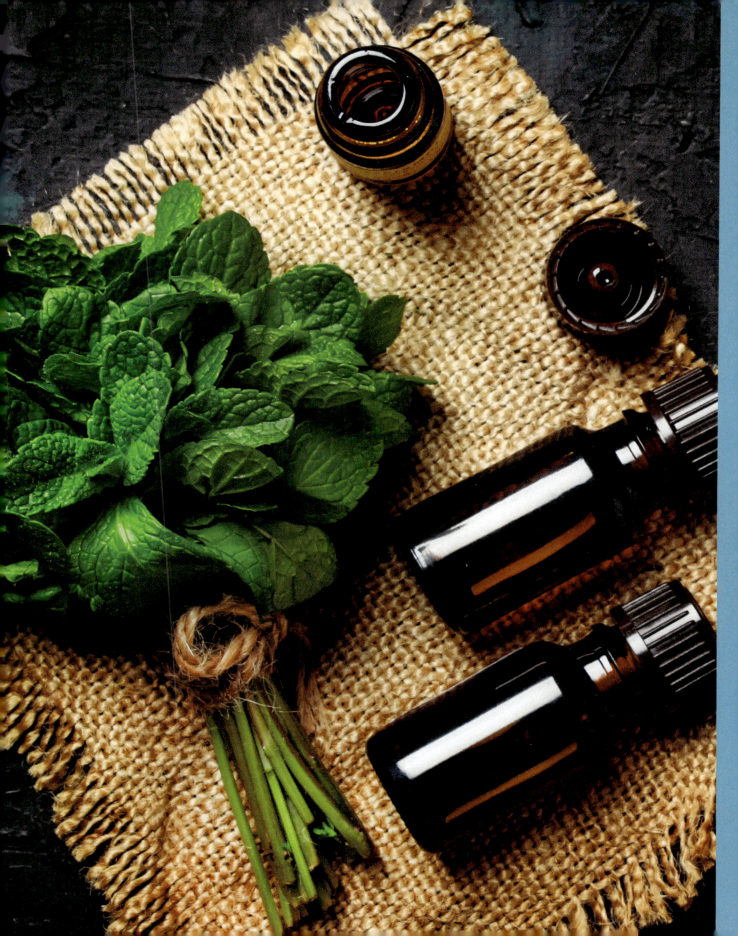

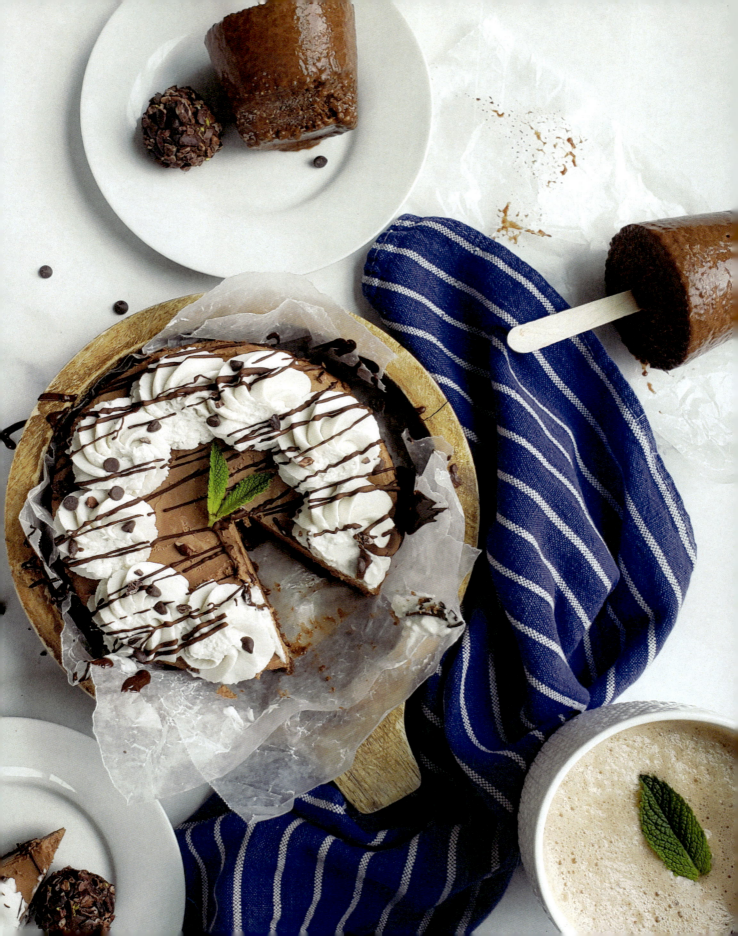

AROMA: *MINTY + COOL* | **FLAVORS:** *MINTY + FRESH*
PAIRS WITH: *CHOCOLATE* | **MAIN USES:** *RESPIRATORY*

Peppermint

MINT CHOCOLATE CHIA PUDDING POPS

2 cans coconut milk
1/4 cup agave or maple syrup
1/2 cup cacao
1/4 cup chia seeds
1 drop Peppermint essential oil

1. Blend the first three ingredients until smooth. Add the Peppermint essential oil at the end.
2. Add 1/4 cup of chia seeds and let the mixture refrigerate for 4 hours or overnight.
3. Portion the soaked chia mixture into popsicle molds and freeze for 4 hours or overnight.

PEPPERMINT HOT CACAO

2 T cacao powder
2 t coconut sugar (optional)
1 drop Peppermint essential oil
pinch pink salt

Mix all ingredients in a mug with a little hot water. Steam or heat your favorite nut milk and pour into the mug. Enjoy!

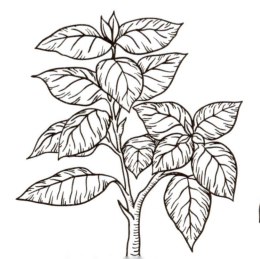
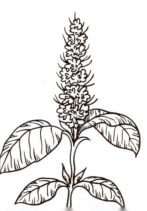

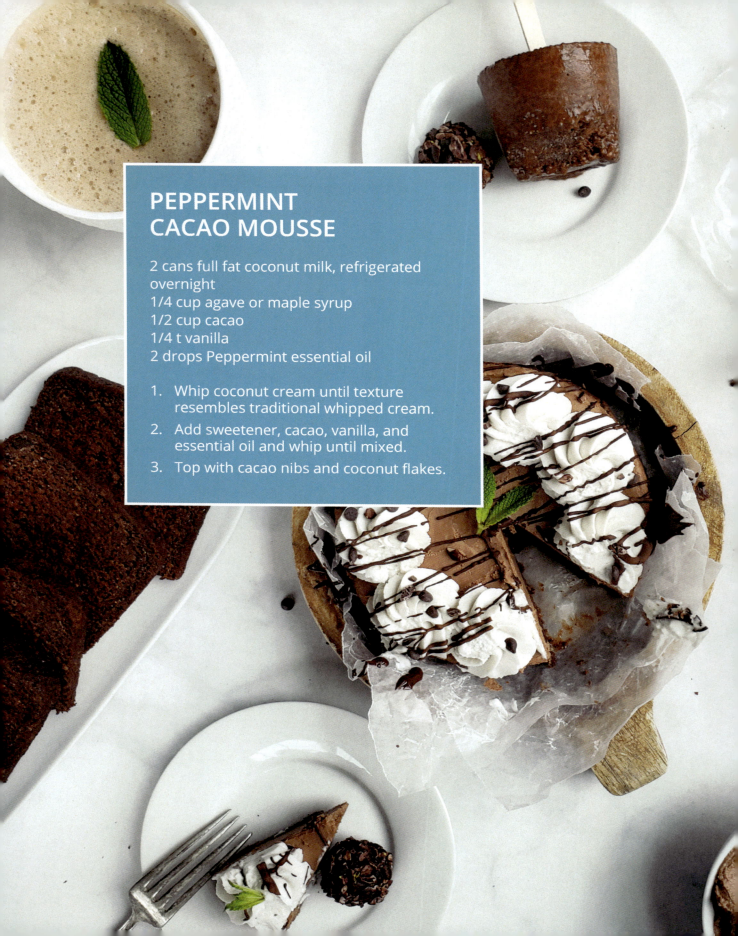

PEPPERMINT CACAO MOUSSE

2 cans full fat coconut milk, refrigerated overnight
1/4 cup agave or maple syrup
1/2 cup cacao
1/4 t vanilla
2 drops Peppermint essential oil

1. Whip coconut cream until texture resembles traditional whipped cream.
2. Add sweetener, cacao, vanilla, and essential oil and whip until mixed.
3. Top with cacao nibs and coconut flakes.

CHOCOLATE PEPPERMINT CHEESECAKE

2 containers Miyoko's vegan cream cheese
3 cans coconut milk—top cream only
1/2 cup melted coconut butter
3/4 cup melted coconut oil
1/2 cup cacao powder
1 cup agave
1/2 t salt
2 t vanilla

1 drop Peppermint essential oil

Combine all ingredients in a high-powered blender. Pour mixture into prepared graham cracker crust. Refrigerate to set for at least 2 hours. Serve with whipped coconut cream and cacao nibs.

CHOCOLATE GLAZED PEPPERMINT BREAD

1/4 cup melted coconut oil
200 mL almond milk
3 T apple cider vinegar
1/2 cup maple syrup
1 t vanilla

1 cup almond flour
1 cup GF flour
1/2 cup cacao powder
pinch salt
1 T baking powder
1/2 t baking soda
2 drops Peppermint essential oil

1 cup dairy free chocolate chips, like Enjoy Life mini chocolate chips
2 T coconut oil
1 drop Peppermint essential oil

1. Combine the liquids in a medium bowl, one that is also large enough to incorporate the dry ingredients.

2. Combine the dry ingredients in a separate bowl and sift them into the bowl with the wet ingredients. Mix gently until just combined.

3. Add the peppermint essential oil just before baking at 325°F for 50-60 minutes.

4. Make a glaze by melting the chocolate chips and coconut oil. Add one drop of peppermint essential oil before drizzling over the top of the cooled chocolate peppermint loaf (taken out of the pan).

5. Refrigerate to set before slicing.

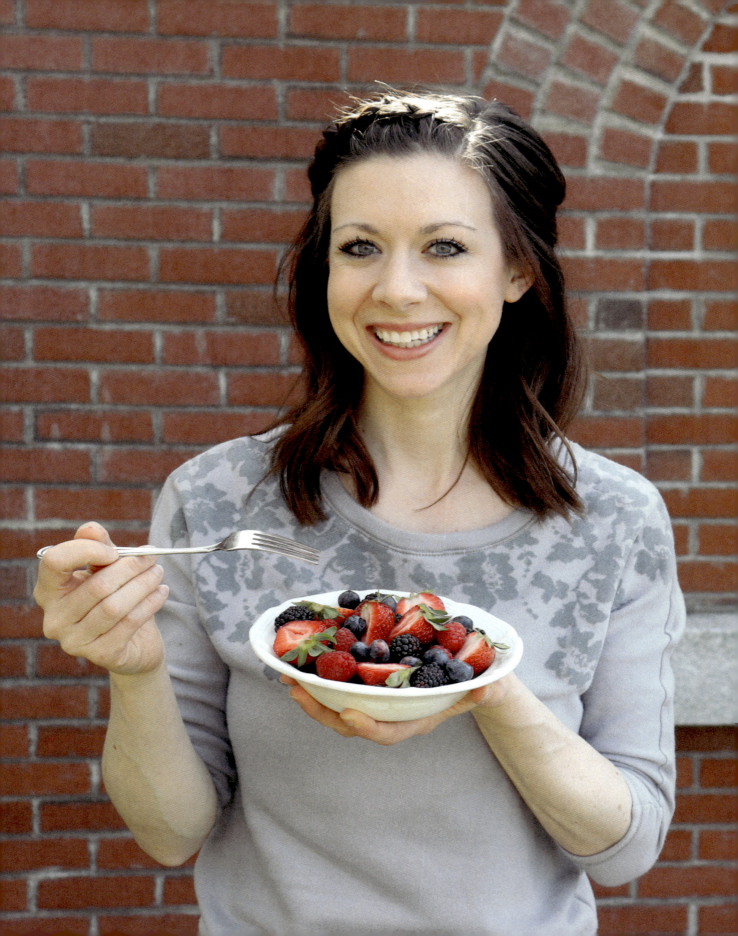

AROMA: SWEET + FRESH | FLAVORS: SWEET + MINTY
PAIRS WITH: BERRY + CACAO | MAIN USES: DIGESTION

Spearmint

MOJITO BERRY SALAD

2 cups total of your favorite berries
2 cups cubed watermelon
1/4 cup lime juice
1 drop Spearmint essential oil

Place fruit in glass or ceramic bowl. Combine lime juice and spearmint oil before adding to the bowl of fruit. Toss gently to combine. Best enjoyed when served immediately.

BLACKBERRY MOJITO

3-4 blackberries
1/2 lime, juiced
1 t coconut sugar

Muddle all ingredients in a glass and top with sparkling water. Add the Spearmint essential oil one toothpick at a time until the desired flavor is reached.

MINT CACAO CHIP NICE CREAM

2-3 T almond milk, or other non-dairy milk
Handful spinach
2 frozen bananas, slightly thawed

1. Blend milk and spinach in a high-powered blender until the milk is green. Add the frozen and slightly thawed bananas and blend slowly until a creamy soft-serve texture is reached. It's helpful if your blender has a tamper to stir the bananas while blending.
2. Stir in 1 drop Spearmint essential oil and cacao nibs before serving.

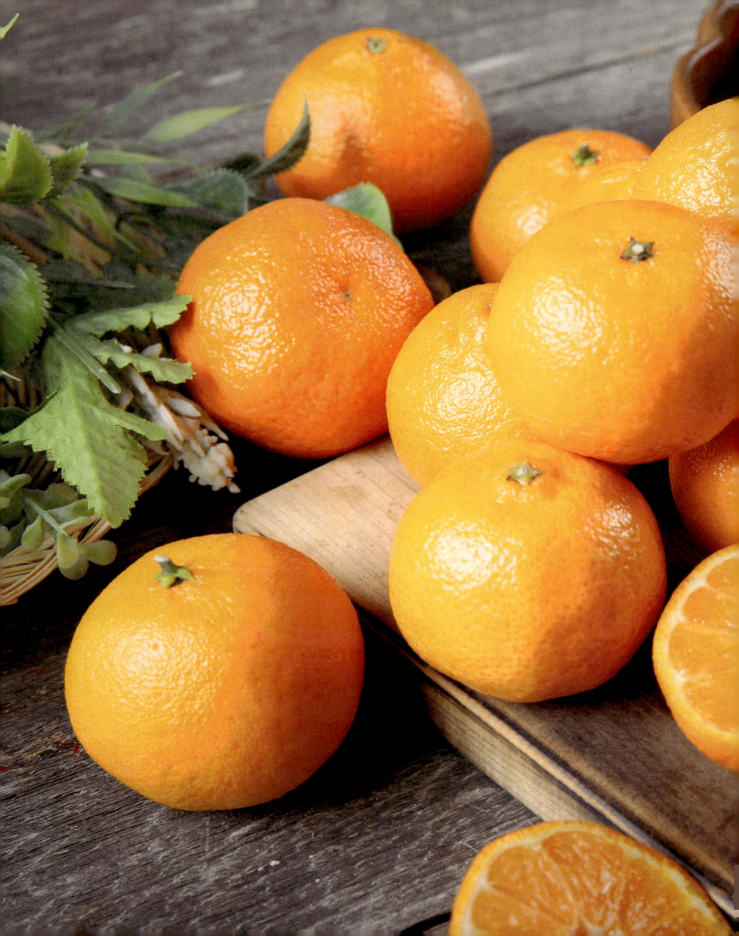

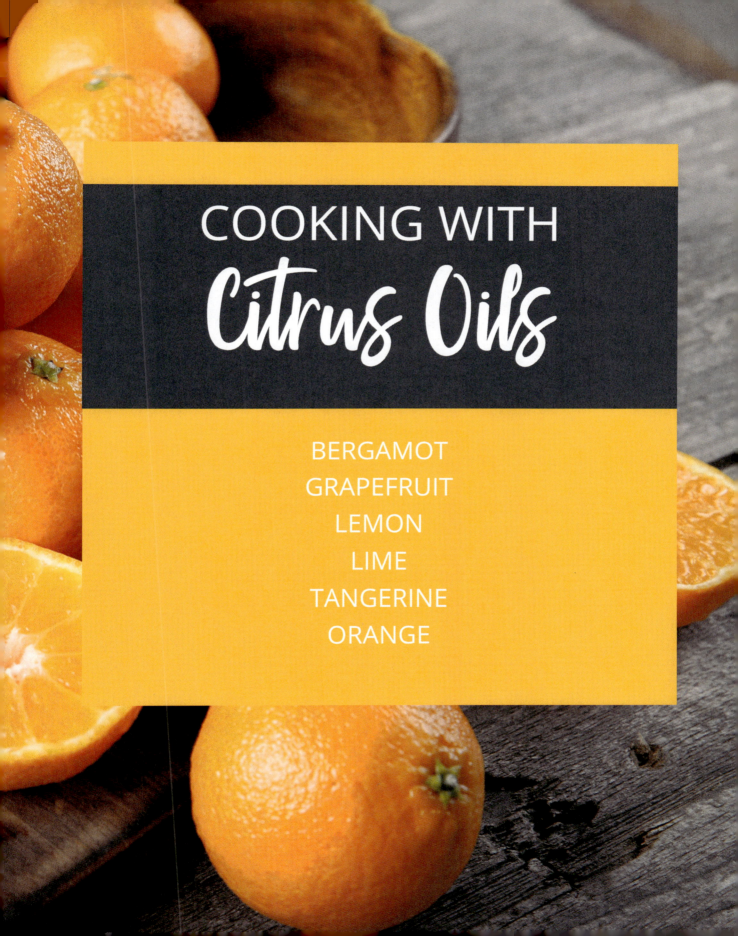

Top Uses of Citrus Oils

Citrus oils provide an uplifting aroma and are helpful in addressing a variety of ailments. In cooking, the essential oil of a citrus fruit would be like using zest or extract. Citrus essential oils will provide a burst of brightness to marinades, dressings, and desserts.

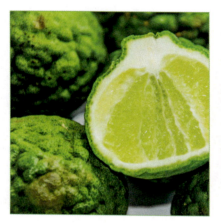

Bergamot

Addictions, insomnia, stress, joint issues and muscle cramps, fungal issues, coughs, infections, bronchitis, acne, oily skin, eczema, psoriasis, appetite loss, self-worth issues, emotional balance

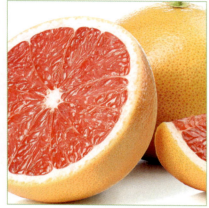

Grapefruit

Weight loss and obesity, breast and uterine issues, progesterone balance, addictions and sugar cravings, oily skin and acne, detoxification, cellulite, lymphatic and kidney toxicity, adrenal fatigue, gallstones and gallbladder support, hangover and jet lag, emotional balance

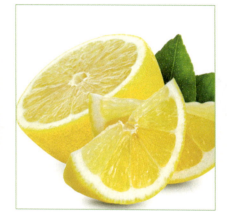

Lemon

Kidney and gallstones, pH issues and lymphatic cleansing, edema and water retention, heartburn and reflux, congestion and mucus, runny nose and allergies, gout, rheumatism, arthritis, liver and kidney detox, degreaser and furniture polish, varicose veins, concentration, emotional balance

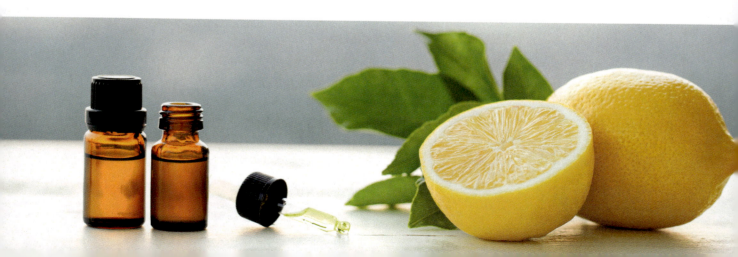

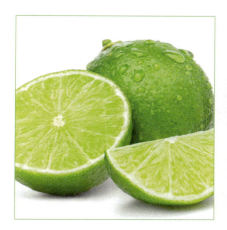 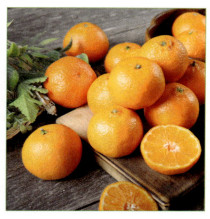 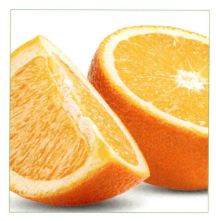

Lime

Sore throat, respiratory, lymph and liver congestion, urinary and digestive issues, memory and clarity, exhaustion and depression, herpes and cold sores, chicken pox, head lice, pain and inflammation, emotional balance

Tangerine

Antioxidant, immune boost, cell protection, sadness and irritability, impulsiveness, sleep issues and anxiety, nervousness, digestive and eliminative disturbances, parasites, overthinking and feeling stuck, edema, cellulite, pocket fat. skin irritations, rashes, burns, dry cracked skin and dandruff, congestion, coughs, asthma, boost metabolism, weight loss, poor circulation, convulsions, achy fatigued muscles and limbs, arthritis and muscle pain, tension, emotional balance

Orange

Insomnia and stress, heartburn and sluggish bowels, scurvy and colds, menopause, depression, fear, anxiety and irritability, lack of energy, creativity and production, concentration, detox and regeneration, digestive upset due to anxiety, emotional balance

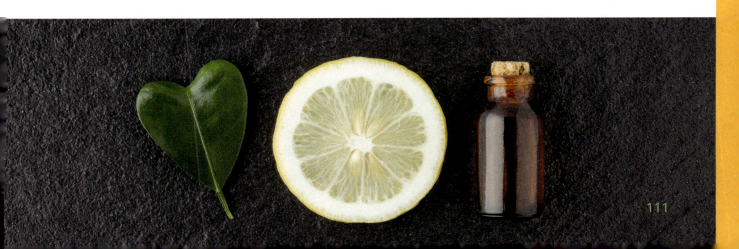

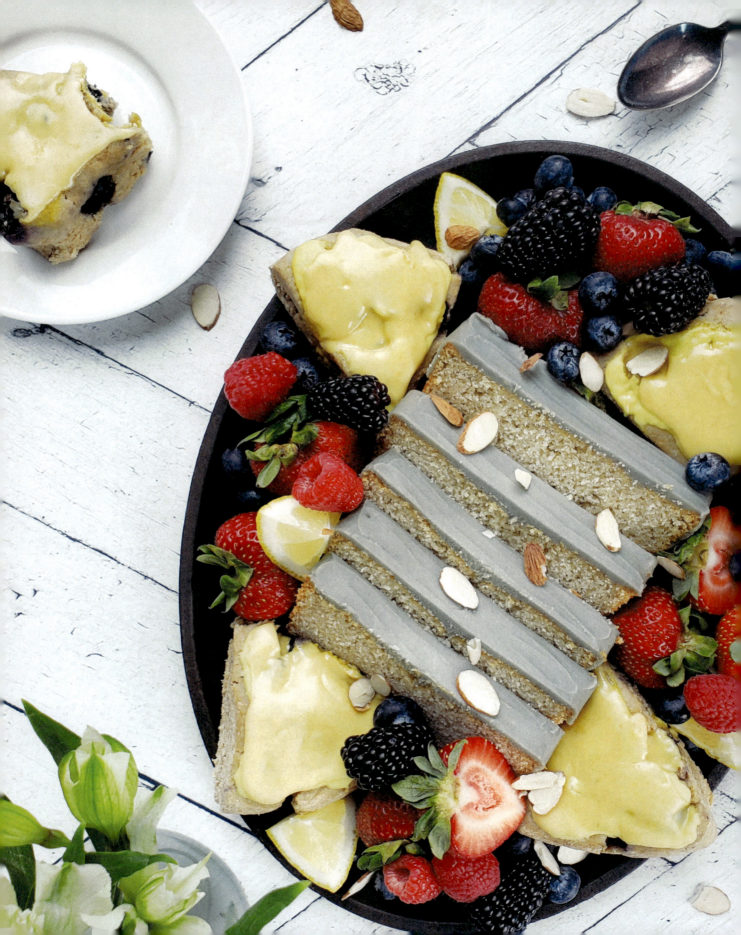

AROMA: SPICE + FLORAL | **FLAVORS:** LEMON + HERBAL
PAIRS WITH: HERBS + WARM SPICES | **MAIN USES:** CALMING

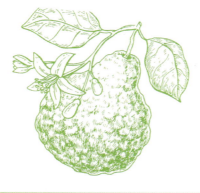

Bergamot

EARL GREY TEA CAKE

1/4 cup melted coconut oil
200 mL almond milk
3 T apple cider vinegar
1/2 cup maple syrup
1 t vanilla

1 1/4 cup almond flour
1 1/4 cup GF flour
pinch salt
1 T baking powder

1/2 t baking soda
3 drops Bergamot essential oil

1. Combine the liquids in a medium bowl, one that is also large enough to incorporate the dry ingredients.
2. Combine the dry ingredients in a separate bowl and sift them into the bowl with the wet ingredients. Mix gently until just combined.
3. Add the bergamot essential oil just before baking at 325°F for 50-60 minutes.
4. Make a glaze by melting 1/4 cup coconut butter. Add one drop of bergamot essential oil, thinning with hot water until thin enough to spread. Optional to add activated charcoal powder to the glaze for the grey color.
5. Once baked, cool the loaf in the pan for 5 minutes before removing to cool completely.
6. Spread the glaze over the top and let it drip down the sides. Refrigerate to set the glaze before slicing and serving.

LEMON, LAVENDER, BERGAMOT SCONES

2 cups oat flour
1/2 cup coconut flour
1/3 cup coconut sugar
1 T baking powder
1 t salt

1/4 cup and 2 T chilled coconut oil

1 cup cold almond milk, unsweetened
2/3 cup frozen blueberries

1 drop each Bergamot, Lemon, Lavender essential oils

1. Combine the dry ingredients in a medium bowl.
2. Cut in the chilled coconut oil and crumble quickly until the texture resembles wet sand.
3. Add the milk and essential oils and stir until just combined. Fold in the frozen blueberries.
4. Transfer the dough onto a floured surface and shape into a large round—about one inch thick.
5. Cut the round into six wedges, place on sheet pan, and brush with coconut milk.
6. Bake at 400°F for 12-15 minutes.
7. Cool completely before glazing.

SCONE GLAZE

1/2 cup powdered sugar
pinch turmeric
1-2 t lemon juice

Whisk glaze ingredients in a small bowl—should be thick!
Spread onto cooled scones and let dry before storing.

EARL GREY TEA

1 hot mug of your favorite plain tea
1 drop Bergamot essential oil
Fresh lemon juice
Honey or maple syrup to taste

Enjoy with scones and good conversation!

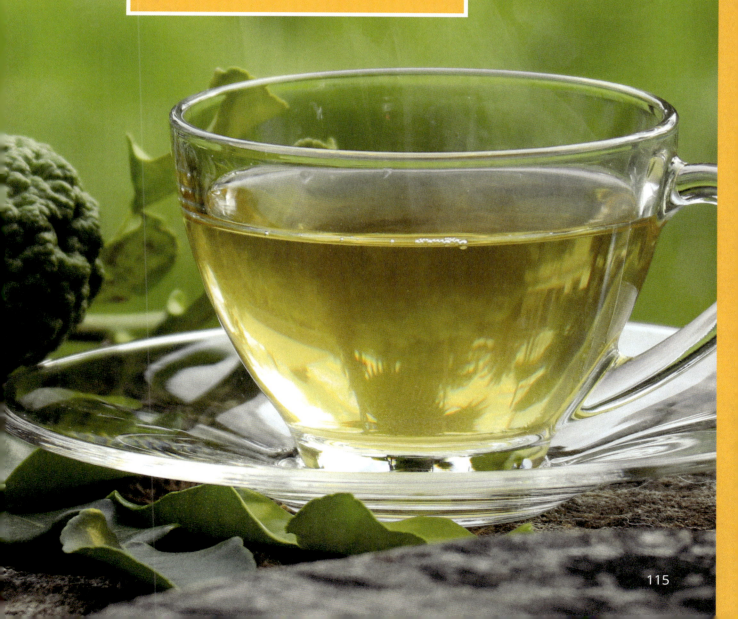

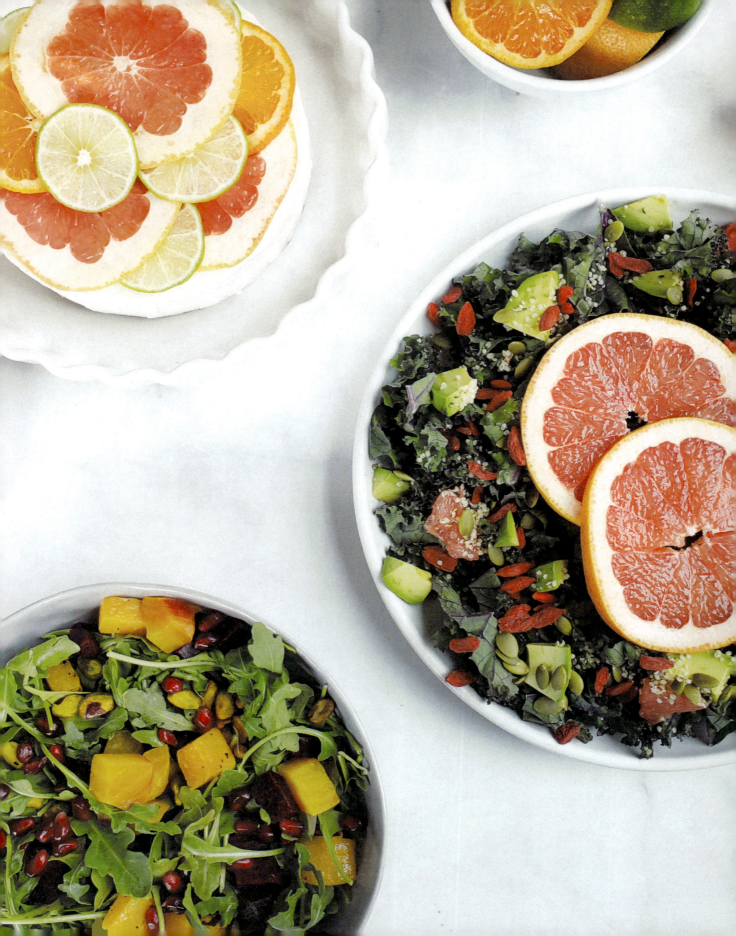

AROMA: *FRUITY + FLORAL* | **FLAVORS:** *SWEET + TART*
PAIRS WITH: *MINT + HERBS* | **MAIN USES:** *METABOLISM*

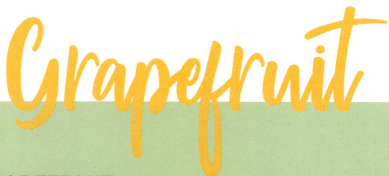

KALE SALAD WITH GRAPEFRUIT, AVOCADO, PUMPKIN SEEDS, AND DIJON GRAPEFRUIT VINAIGRETTE

Dressing:
1 T Dijon mustard
1 T white wine vinegar
1 t maple syrup
1 drop Grapefruit essential oil

Salad:
1 head kale, chopped
1 grapefruit, peeled and cut into segments
1 avocado, diced
1/4 cup pumpkin seeds

1. In a medium bowl, mix dressing ingredients. Whisk in 1 T avocado or olive oil to complete dressing.
2. To the bowl add chopped kale and massage for about 5 minutes, until the leaves become tender.
3. Add grapefruit pieces, diced avocado, and pumpkin seeds. Sprinkle with hemp seeds or roasted chickpeas for added protein.

ROASTED BEET SALAD WITH GRAPEFRUIT VINAIGRETTE

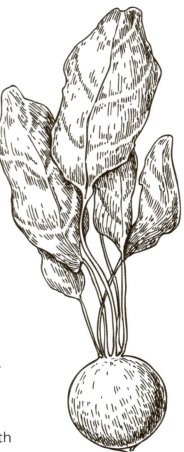

Dressing:
1 T Dijon mustard
1 T white wine vinegar
1 t maple syrup
1 drop Grapefruit essential oil

Salad:
2-4 beets, cubed
1-2 red onions
1-2 sweet potatoes, diced
1 8oz container arugula
1/4 cup pistachios
Local honey

1. In a medium bowl, mix 1 T Dijon mustard, 1 T white wine vinegar, 1 t maple syrup, and 1 drop Grapefruit essential oil. Whisk in 1 T avocado or olive oil to complete dressing.
2. Cube beets and roast in oven with sliced onions and diced sweet potato until tender.
3. Toss in a little olive oil if you like here, and season with a pinch of Himalayan pink salt.
4. Add arugula or your favorite green to the dressing bowl along with the roasted veggies. Top with pistachios and a drizzle of local honey.

FRUIT SALAD DRESSING

1. In a large bowl, combine seasonal fruits like berries, stone fruit, tropical fruit, etc.
2. In a small bowl, mix equal parts local honey, orange juice or lemon juice, and a drop of Grapefruit essential oil.
3. Drizzle over fruit and toss to combine before enjoying.

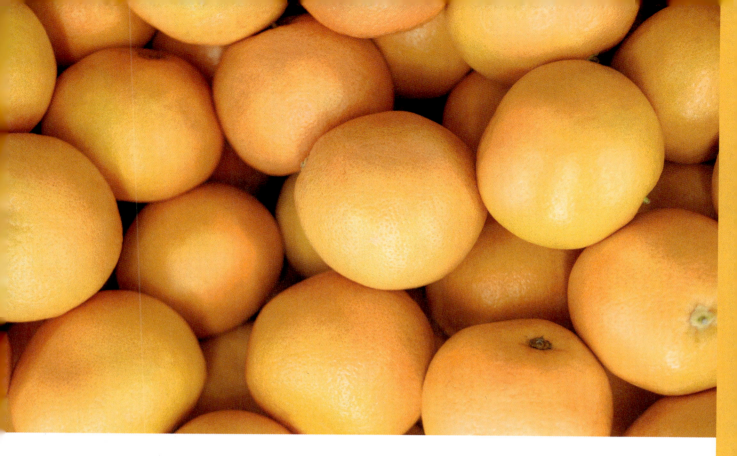

CITRUS BURST CHEESECAKE

2 containers Miyoko's vegan cream cheese
3 cans coconut milk—top cream only
1/2 cup melted coconut butter
3/4 cup melted coconut oil
1 T lemon juice
1 cup agave
1/2 t salt
2 t vanilla
2 drops each Grapefruit, Lime, Tangerine essential oils

Combine all ingredients in a high-powered blender. Pour mixture into prepared graham cracker crust. Refrigerate to set for at least 2 hours. Serve with fresh lime wedges and toasted coconut flakes.

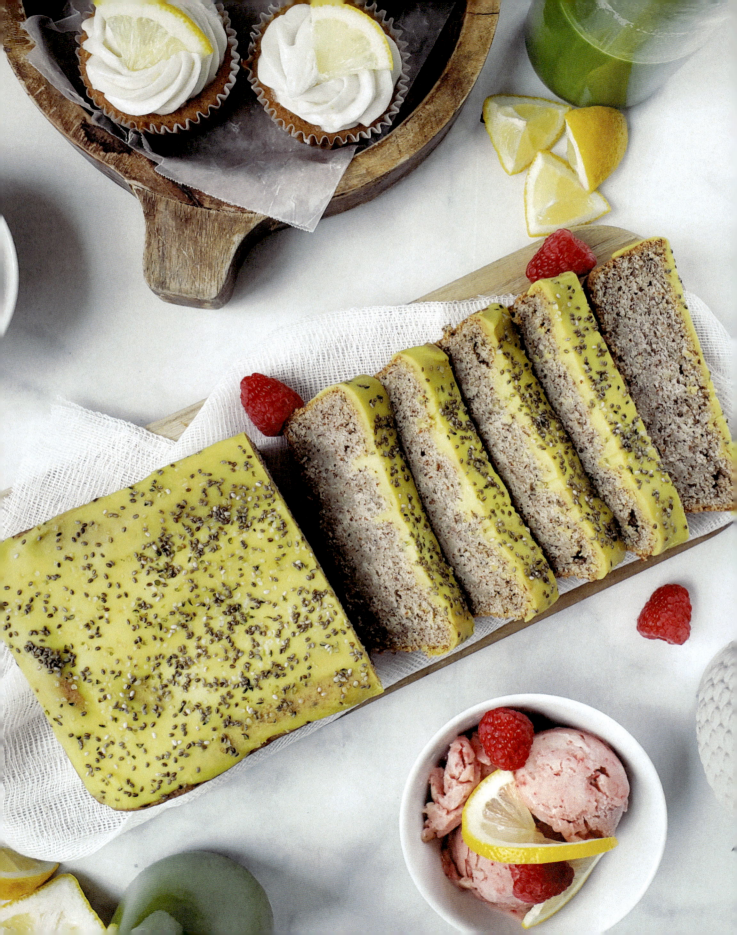

AROMA: *FRESH + BRIGHT* | **FLAVORS:** *SWEET + SHARP*
PAIRS WITH: *HERBS + FRUIT* | **MAIN USES:** *CLEANSING*

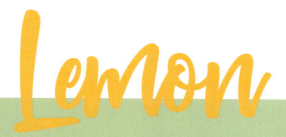

LEMON CHIA BREAD

1/4 cup melted coconut oil
200 mL almond milk
3 T apple cider vinegar
1/2 cup maple syrup
1 t vanilla

1 1/4 cup almond flour
1 1/4 cup GF flour
pinch salt
1 T baking powder
1/2 t baking soda

3 drops Lemon essential oil
1 T each chia seeds and hemp seeds

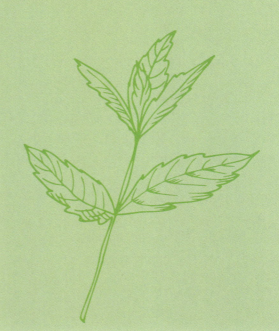

1. Combine the liquids in a medium bowl, one that is also large enough to incorporate the dry ingredients.
2. Combine the dry ingredients in a separate bowl and sift them into the bowl with the wet ingredients. Mix gently until just combined.
3. Add the Lemon essential oil just before baking at 325°F for 50-60 minutes.
4. Make a glaze by melting 1/4 cup coconut butter. Add 1-2 T maple syrup and one drop of Lemon essential oil, thinning with hot water until thin enough to spread. Optional to add a pinch of turmeric powder to the glaze for the yellow color.
5. Once baked, cool the loaf in the pan for 5 minutes before removing to cool completely.
6. Spread the glaze over the top and let it drip down the sides. Top with additional chia seeds. Refrigerate to set the glaze before slicing and serving.

LEMONY PASTA WITH SPINACH AND OLIVES

1 yellow onion, diced
1 clove fresh pressed garlic
1 t white wine vinegar

1 box GF pasta
2 cups water
1/4 cup nutritional yeast
1/4 t fresh cracked pepper

Handfuls of fresh spinach or kale
Chopped olives, your favorite kind

1. In a medium pot, saute the onion until fragrant—about 4 minutes.
2. Add garlic and cook for 1 minute more. Deglaze the pot with white wine vinegar, or regular white wine (something dry).
3. Add the pasta, water, nutritional yeast, and pepper to the pot. Stir to combine before turning up the heat to bring to a low boil.
4. Reduce heat to low and simmer, with a lid, until pasta is cooked—about 5 minutes.
5. Add tons of fresh spinach or baby kale and the chopped olives. Continue cooking until greens are wilted and pasta is cooked.
6. Add one drop of Lemon essential oil to a small dish with 1 T extra virgin olive oil and 1 t fresh lemon juice to dilute the flavor for even distribution.
7. Pour over pasta, season with salt to taste, and garnish with fresh parsley, vegan parmesan cheese, or fresh cracked pepper.

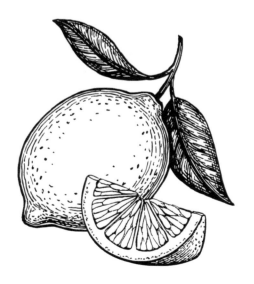

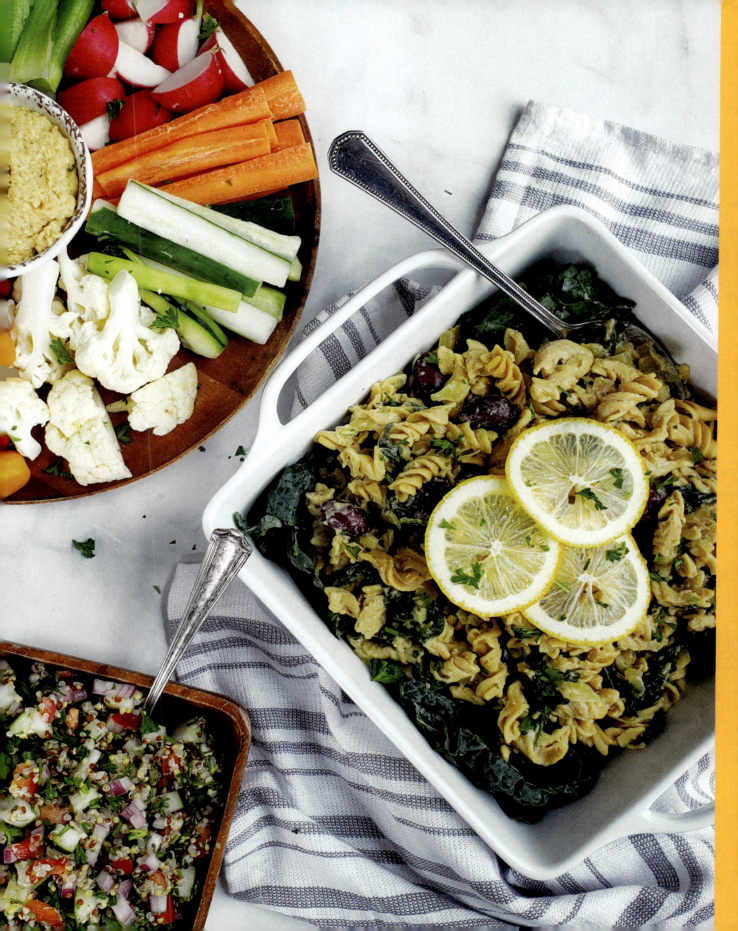

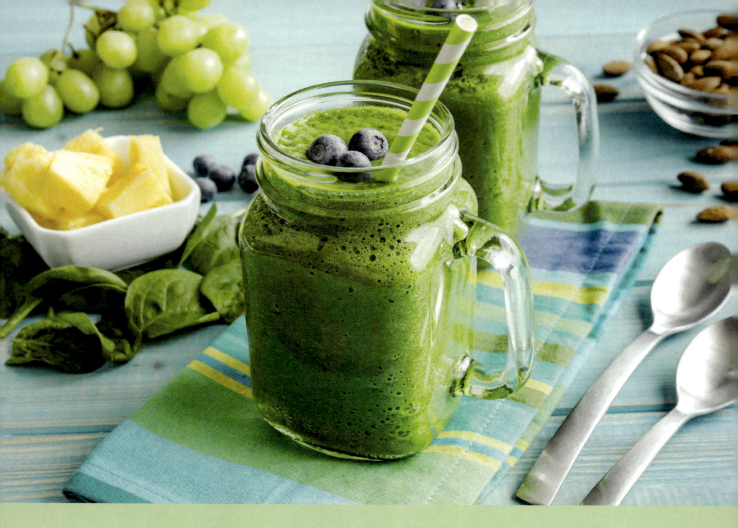

GREEN DETOX SMOOTHIE

8 oz coconut or almond milk
2 cups greens
1 banana
1/4 cup parsley
2 drops Lemon essential oil
1 cup blueberries

Blend all ingredients in a high-powered blender, adding essential oil toward the end.

LEMON HERB VINAIGRETTE

2 T extra virgin olive oil
2 T apple cider vinaigrette
2 T lemon juice
1 drop Lemon essential oil
1 toothpick Oregano essential oil

Whisk in bowl before tossing with Quinoa Tabbouleh.

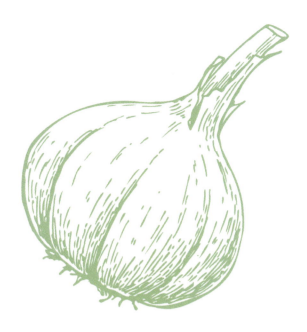

LEMON GARLIC HUMMUS

2 15-oz cans chickpeas, drained and rinsed
1 T fresh garlic
2 T tahini
1/2 t salt
1 t lemon juice
1 drop Lemon essential oil

Mix well in a food processor, adding the essential oil in the last few seconds of blending.

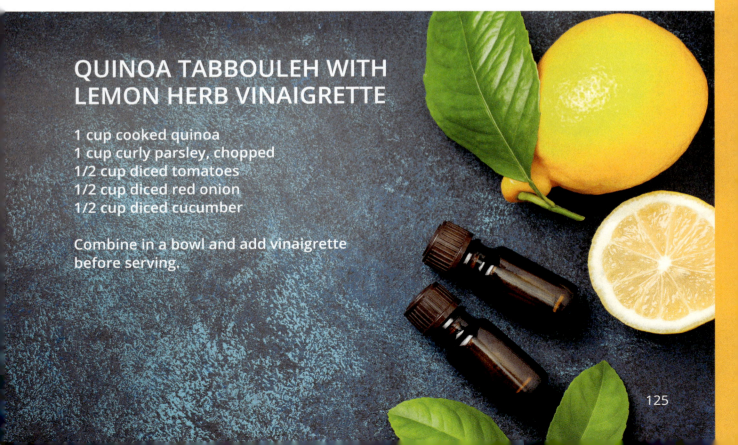

QUINOA TABBOULEH WITH LEMON HERB VINAIGRETTE

1 cup cooked quinoa
1 cup curly parsley, chopped
1/2 cup diced tomatoes
1/2 cup diced red onion
1/2 cup diced cucumber

Combine in a bowl and add vinaigrette before serving.

LEMON BURST CUPCAKES

1 2/3 cups almond milk
1 1/2 t apple cider vinegar
1 T lemon juice
1/3 cup applesauce
1 t vanilla

3 1/4 cup almond flour
1 cup potato starch
1/3 cup arrowroot
1 1/2 cups coconut sugar
1 1/2 t baking powder
1 1/2 t baking soda
1/2 t salt

4 drops Lemon essential oil
1 lemon, zested (optional)

1. Combine almond milk and apple cider vinegar in a measuring cup and let sit for 5 minutes to curdle the milk.
2. Add the lemon juice, applesauce and vanilla to a bowl along with the curdled milk.
3. Mix the dry ingredients in a large bowl. Add the wet ingredients and stir until no lumps remain.
4. Stir in the Lemon essential oil and optional zest before portioning the batter into a sprayed or lined cupcake pan.
5. Bake at 350°F for 20 minutes, or until a toothpick comes out clean.
6. Cool in the pan for a few minutes before removing to cool completely.
7. Frost with a batch of vanilla frosting (see page 133), adding 1/2 t lemon juice, 2-3 drops Lemon essential oil, and 1/4 t turmeric powder for color.

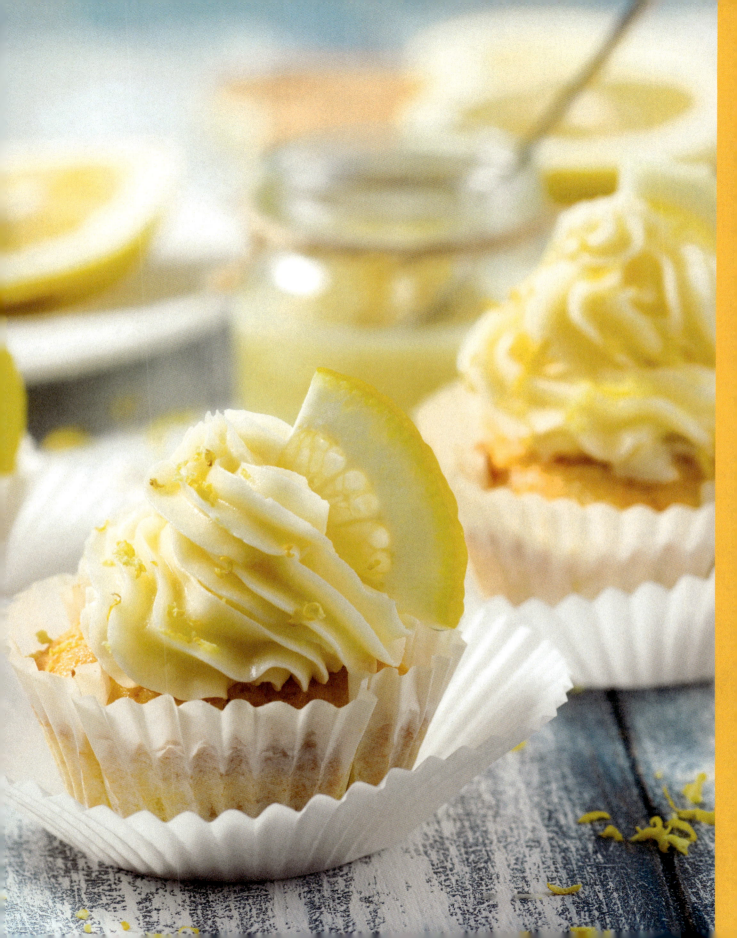

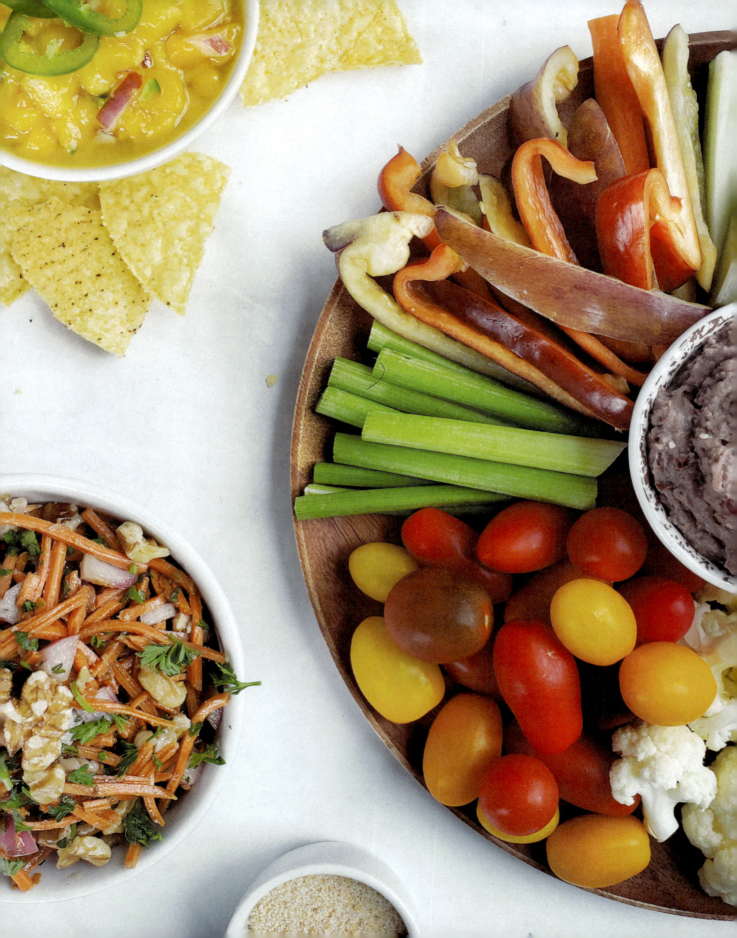

AROMA: *TART + SWEET* | **FLAVORS:** *TANGY + SWEET*
PAIRS WITH: *COCONUT, MINT + HERBS* | **MAIN USES:** *IMMUNITY*

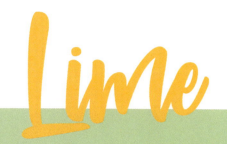

Lime

CARROT SALAD WITH LIME AND CILANTRO

2 cups shredded carrots
1/2 cup chopped walnuts
1/4 cup minced red onion
1/4 cup fresh parsley

In a bowl, combine 2 T olive oil, 1 T apple cider vinegar, 2 drops Lime and 1 drop Cilantro essential oil, and 1 t maple syrup. Add above ingredients and stir to coat.

MANGO LIME SALSA

2 mangoes, diced
2-3 T minced red onion
1/2 jalapeno, seeded and minced
1 T lime juice
1/4 t salt
1 drop Lime essential oil

Combine all ingredients in a bowl and enjoy with chips or added to a power bowl or salad.

BLACK BEAN LIME HUMMUS

2 15-oz cans black beans, drained and rinsed
1 T tahini
1/2 t salt
1 t lime juice
1/2 t cumin
1 drop each Lime and Cilantro essential oils

Mix well in a food processor, adding the oils in the last few seconds of blending.

CITRUS SEASONING SALT

3 T Himalayan pink salt
1 drop each Lime, Lemon, Tangerine essential oils
1 T granulated garlic
1 T dry mustard

Use with grilled veggies, in sauces or dressings, or added to grain dishes.

COCONUT LIME CHEESECAKE

2 containers Miyoko's vegan cream cheese
3 cans coconut milk—top cream only
1/2 cup melted coconut butter
3/4 cup melted coconut oil
1 T lemon juice
1 cup agave
1/2 t salt
2 t vanilla
3 drops Lime essential oil

Combine all ingredients in a high-powered blender. Pour mixture into prepared graham cracker crust. Refrigerate to set for at least 2 hours. Serve with fresh lime wedges and toasted coconut flakes.

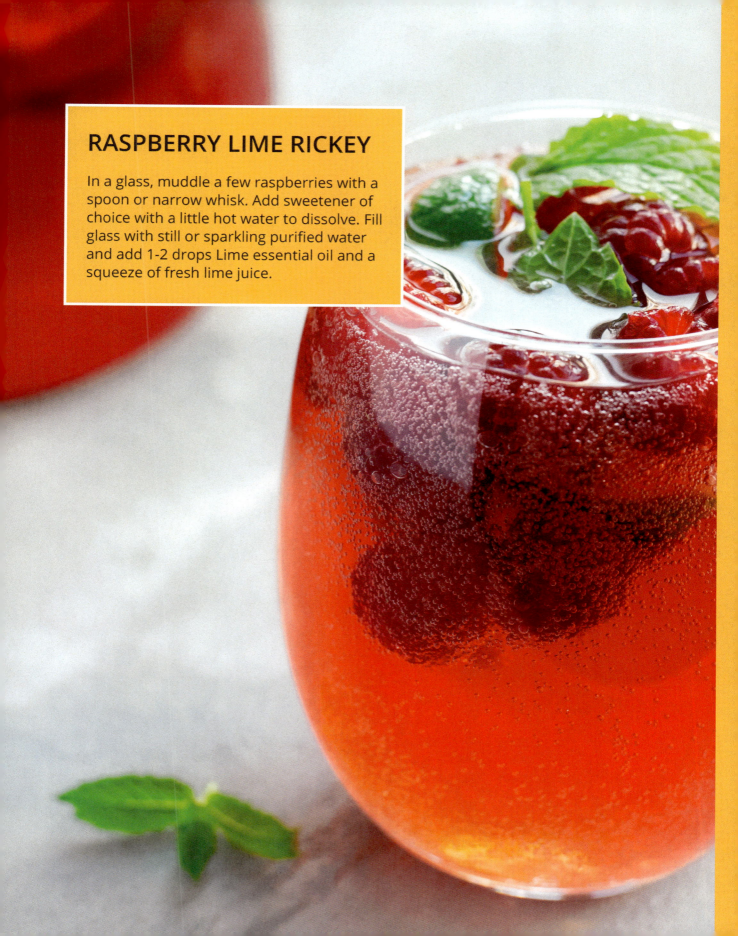

RASPBERRY LIME RICKEY

In a glass, muddle a few raspberries with a spoon or narrow whisk. Add sweetener of choice with a little hot water to dissolve. Fill glass with still or sparkling purified water and add 1-2 drops Lime essential oil and a squeeze of fresh lime juice.

LIME CUPCAKES

1 2/3 cups almond milk
1 1/2 t apple cider vinegar
1 T lime juice
1/3 cup applesauce
1 t vanilla

3 1/4 cup almond flour
1 cup potato starch
1/3 cup arrowroot
1 1/2 cups coconut sugar
1 1/2 t baking powder
1 1/2 t baking soda
1/2 t salt

4 drops Lime essential oil
1 lime, zested (optional)

1. Combine almond milk and apple cider vinegar in a measuring cup and let sit for 5 minutes to curdle the milk.
2. Add the lime juice, applesauce and vanilla to a bowl along with the curdled milk.
3. Mix the dry ingredients in a large bowl. Add the wet ingredients and stir until no lumps remain.
4. Stir in the Lime essential oil and optional zest before portioning the batter into a sprayed or lined cupcake pan.
5. Bake at 350°F for 20 minutes, or until a toothpick comes out clean.
6. Cool in the pan for a few minutes before removing to cool completely.
7. Frost with a batch of vanilla frosting, adding 1/2 t lime juice, 2-3 drops Lime essential oil, and lime zest or natural green food color (optional).

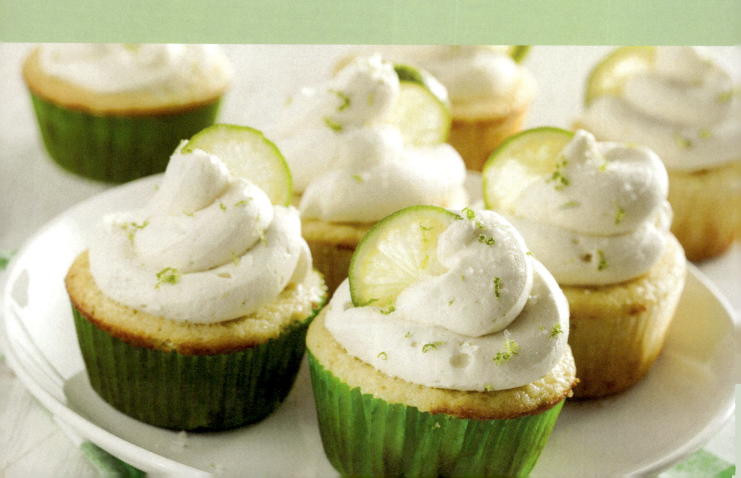

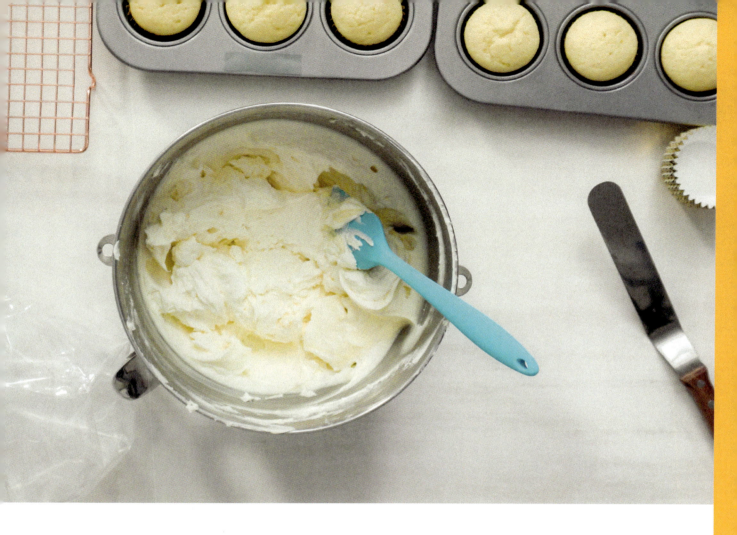

VANILLA FROSTING

1 cup coconut oil, firm but not cold

2 cans coconut milk, chilled, and use the hardened cream only

1/4 cup agave
1 t vanilla
1/4 cup melted coconut butter

1. Whip the coconut oil with electric mixer, using the whisk attachment. Be careful not to over mix and melt the oil.
2. Add the coconut cream, the hardened portion from the top half of the can. Save the milk for another use.
3. Whip to incorporate—the mixture may start to break, so add slowly and scrape the sides regularly.
4. Add the agave and vanilla, then turn on the mixer and add the melted coconut butter while mixing. This step brings the frosting together. More coconut butter may be needed.
5. Add the desired essential oils, and a little of the same citrus juice, toward the end of mixing.
6. Optional to add natural food color before frosting cupcakes.

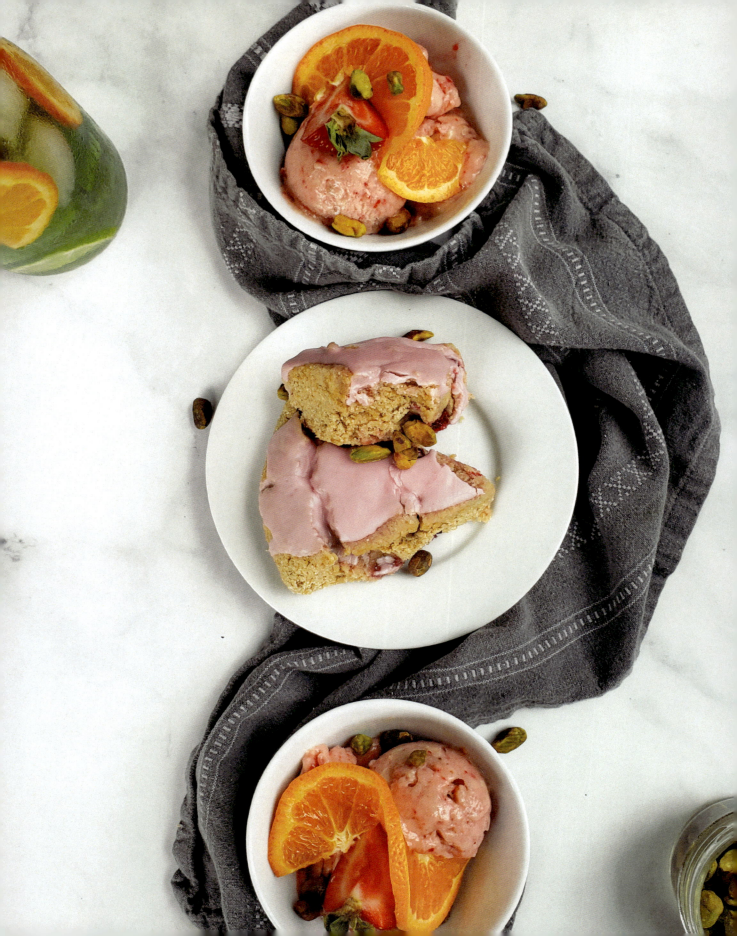

AROMA: *TANGY + SWEET* | **FLAVORS:** *BRIGHT + SWEET*
PAIRS WITH: *VINEGARS + BERRIES* | **MAIN USES:** *IMMUNITY*

Tangerine

CREAMSICLE NICE CREAM

2 frozen bananas
3-4 frozen strawberries slightly thawed
2-3 T almond milk, or other non-dairy milk

1. Blend in a high-powered blender until creamy like soft-serve ice cream. It's helpful to use the tamper while blending to help move the bananas.
2. Stir in 1 drop Tangerine essential oil before serving.

LIMEADE WITH LOCAL HONEY

In a glass, mix honey with a little hot water to melt. Fill glass with still or sparkling purified water and add 1-2 drops Lime essential oil and a squeeze of fresh lime juice or apple cider vinegar (for tartness).

TANGERINE ROASTED PISTACHIOS

2 cups pistachios
1/4 t avocado oil
3 drops Tangerine essential oil
1/4 t Himalayan pink salt

1. Roast the pistachios dry at 250°F for 4-5 minutes.
2. Mix the avocado oil and essential oil in a small bowl before tossing with the pistachios.
3. Season with salt to taste. Optional to add a drizzle of honey.

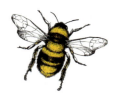

STRAWBERRY TANGERINE SCONES

2 cups oat flour
1/2 cup coconut flour
1/3 cup coconut sugar
1 T baking powder
1 t salt

1/4 cup + 2 T chilled coconut oil
1 cup cold almond milk, unsweetened

2/3 cup fresh or frozen strawberries
2 drops Tangerine essential oil

1. Combine the dry ingredients in a medium bowl.
2. Cut in the chilled coconut oil and crumble quickly until the texture resembles wet sand.
3. Add the milk and essential oils and stir until just combined. Fold in the strawberries.
4. Transfer the dough onto a floured surface and shape into a large round—about one inch thick.
5. Cut the round into six wedges, place on sheet pan, and brush with coconut milk.
6. Bake at 400°F for 12-15 minutes.
7. Cool completely before glazing.

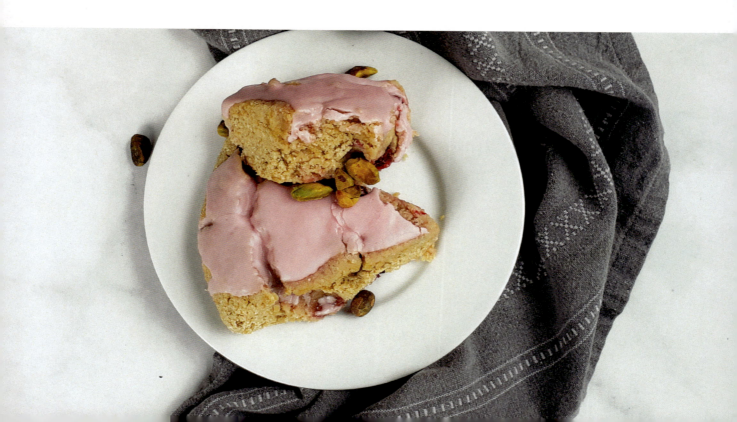

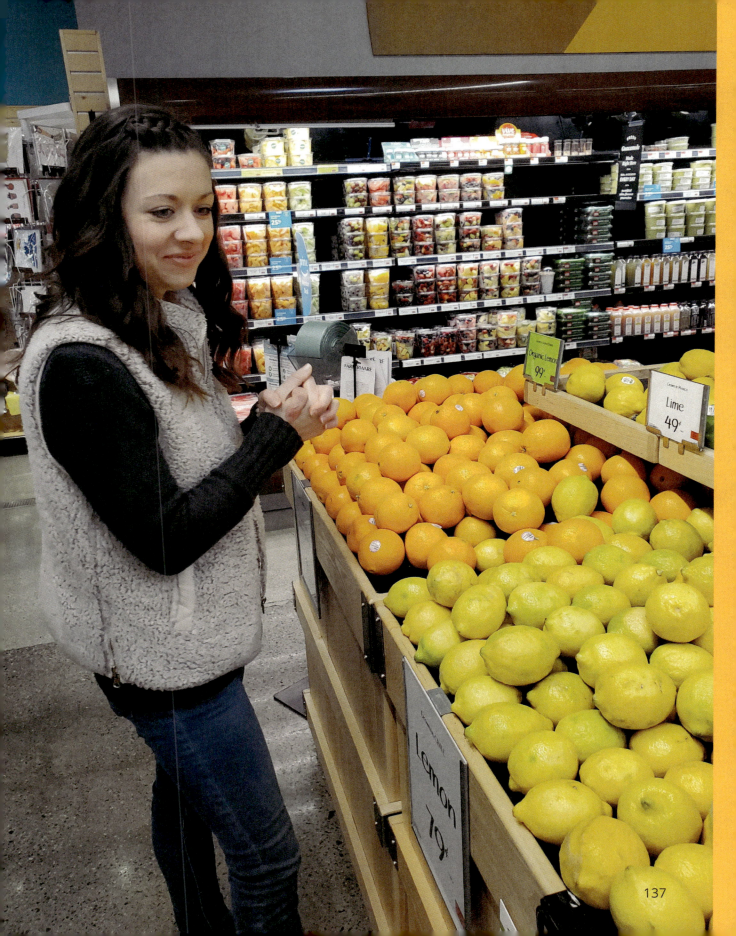

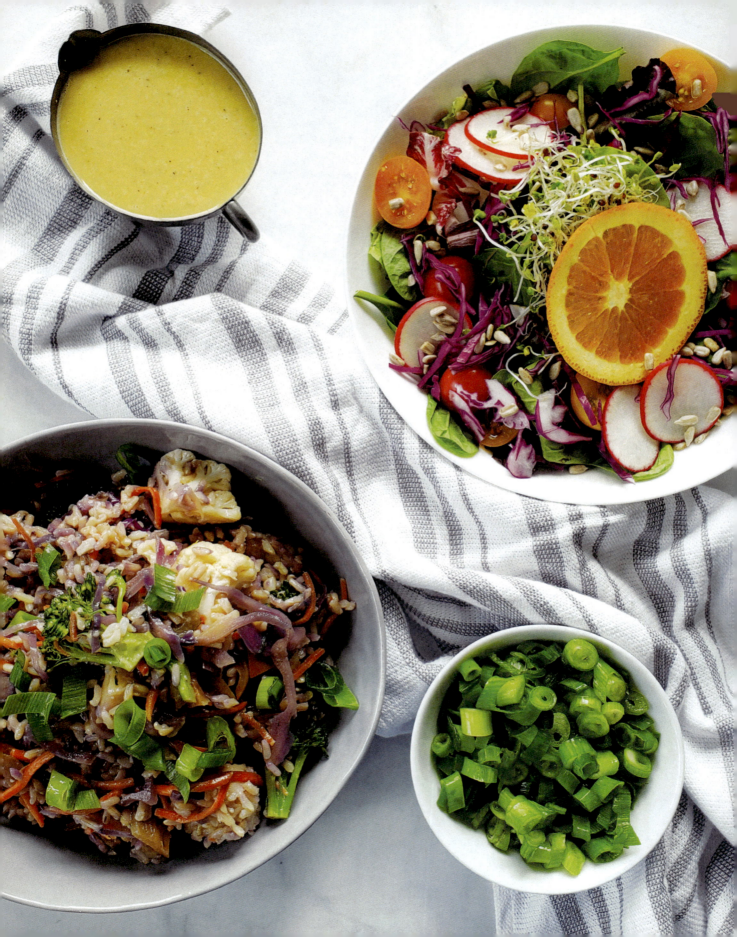

AROMA: *SWEET + FRESH* | **FLAVORS:** *LIGHT + TART*
PAIRS WITH: *ASIAN CUISINE* | **MAIN USES:** *CLEANSING*

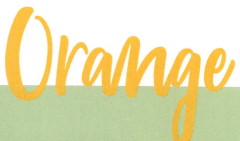

HONEY ORANGE ROASTED ALMONDS

2 cups almonds
1/4 t avocado oil
1/4 t Himalayan pink salt
3 drops Orange essential oil
1 T local honey

Roast nuts plain at 250°F for 12-15 minutes. Combine oils in bowl before adding roasted nuts. Season with salt to taste and return to oven to bake for 5-8 minutes.

SWEET AND SOUR STIR FRY

1. Make stir fry as usual, using your favorite veggies and proteins.
2. In a small bowl, combine tamari and water in a 2:1 ratio.
3. Add fresh pressed garlic, 2 drops Orange essential oil, a splash of maple syrup, 1/4 cup pineapple juice, 1/4 cup rice vinegar, 1 T ketchup, and a little arrowroot, tapioca starch, or cornstarch to help thicken. Pour sauce into the center of the stir fry pan or wok and cook for a few minutes.
4. Continue cooking until sauce has thickened and coated veggies to your liking.
5. Make it as saucy as you like—I prefer to have extra so there is enough to cover the rice or quinoa.

BLUEBERRY MUFFIN SMOOTHIE

8 oz almond or oat milk
1 cup blueberries
1 banana
1 cup spinach
1/4 cup oats
Dash cinnamon
1 drop Orange essential oil

Blend in a high-powered blender until smooth, adding essential oil toward the end.

ORANGE CHOCOLATE TRUFFLES

1 can coconut milk, refrigerated overnight—use top cream only
1 bag dairy free chocolate chips
2 drops Orange essential oil

Melt coconut cream and chocolate chips until smooth. Stir in essential oil and refrigerate until firm but still soft enough to scoop into truffles. Roll in cacao powder, coconut flakes, chopped nuts or a mixture!

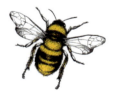

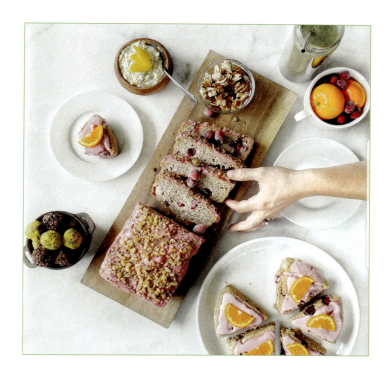

CRANBERRY ORANGE BREAD

1/4 cup melted coconut oil
200 mL almond milk
3 T apple cider vinegar
1/2 cup maple syrup
1 t vanilla

1 1/4 cup almond flour
1 1/4 cup GF flour
Pinch salt
1 T baking powder
1/2 t baking soda

4 drops Orange essential oil
1 cup frozen cranberries

1/4 cup melted coconut butter
2 T agave
1/4 t vanilla
2 drops Orange essential oil

1. Combine the liquids in a medium bowl, one that is also large enough to incorporate the dry ingredients.
2. Combine the dry ingredients in a separate bowl and sift them into the bowl with the wet ingredients. Mix gently until just combined.
3. Add the Orange essential oil just before baking at 325°F for 50-60 minutes.
4. Make a glaze by melting 1/4 cup coconut butter. Add 1-2 T maple syrup and one drop of Orange essential oil, thinning with hot water until thin enough to spread. Optional to add natural food color, or 1/2 t beet juice.
5. Once baked, cool the loaf in the pan for 5 minutes before removing to cool completely.
6. Spread the glaze over the top and let it drip down the sides. Top with chopped walnuts. Refrigerate to set the glaze before slicing and serving.

TROPICAL ORANGE MOUSSE

2 cans full fat coconut milk
1 T maple syrup
1/4 cup fresh mango, diced small
1/4 cup fresh pineapple, diced small
2 drops Orange essential oil

1. Chill coconut milk for 2 hours. Scoop top cream only into a bowl and whisk with hand or stand mixer until fluffy.
2. Add maple syrup and whip another few seconds. Fold in diced fruit and essential oil.

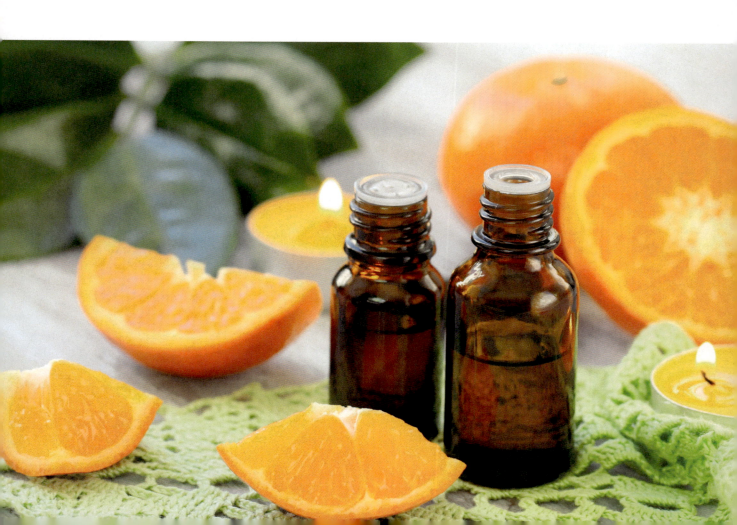

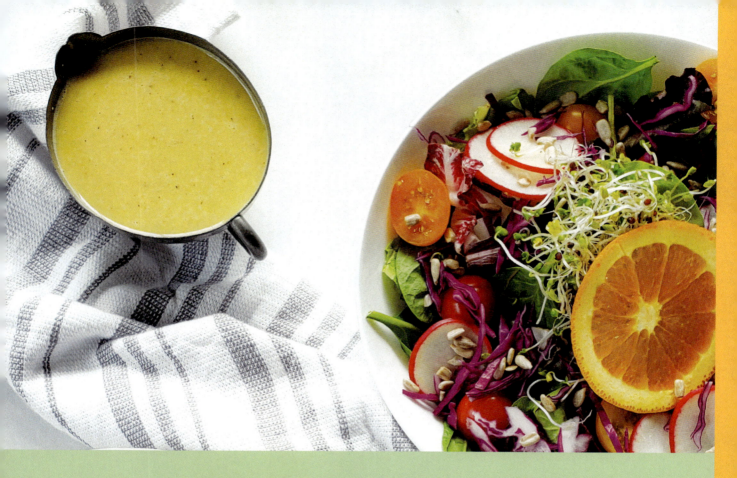

ORANGE VINAIGRETTE

1 small shallot
1 clove garlic
1/2 cup orange juice
2 T white balsamic vinegar
1 T maple syrup
1/4 t salt
1/4 t pepper
1/2 t Dijon mustard
1/2 t lemon juice
1 T local honey
1/4 cup extra-virgin olive oil
1 drop Orange essential oil

1. Toss everything except essential oil in a high-powered blender and blend until smooth.
2. Add essential oil in at the very end before transferring to a glass bottle.
3. Serve on a superfood salad, use as a marinade, or over a power bowl.

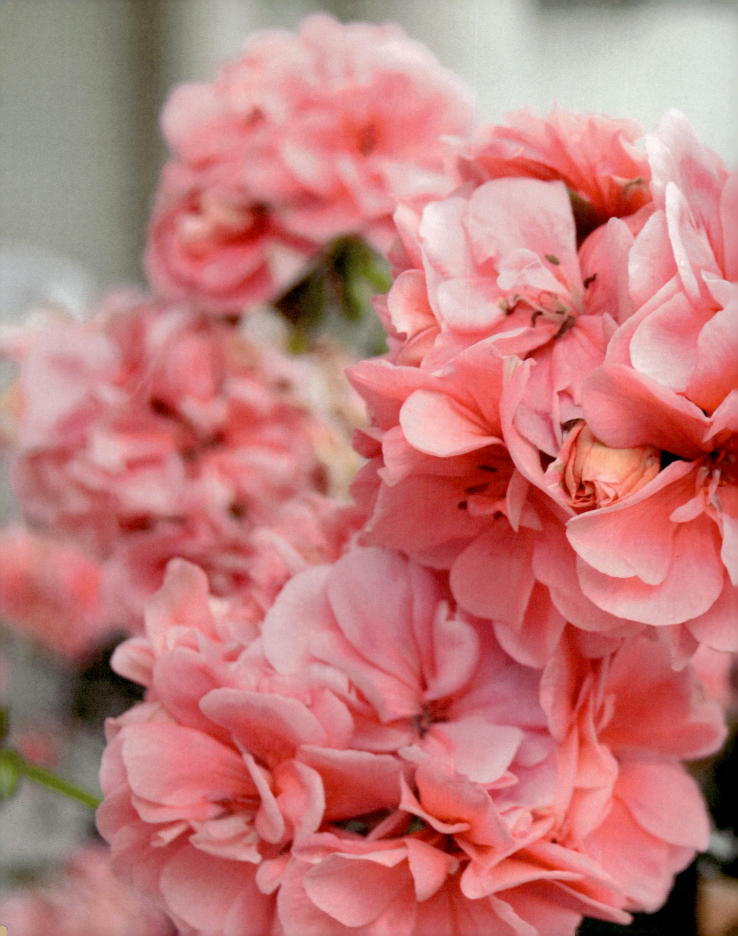

COOKING WITH
Floral Oils

GERANIUM
LAVENDER

Top Uses of Floral Oils

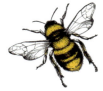

When used in cooking, floral oils add a level of timeless sophistication and elegance. They are also very handy to have readily available in your cupboard for burns and cuts.

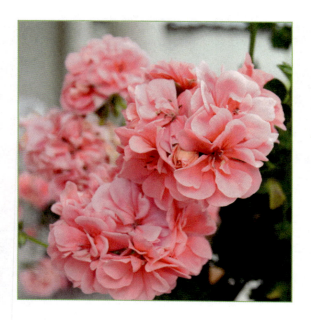

Geranium

Liver, gallbladder, pancreas and kidney issues, blood issues and bleeding, cuts and wounds, PMS and hormone balancing, low libido, dry or oily hair and skin, moisturizer, body odor, emotional balance

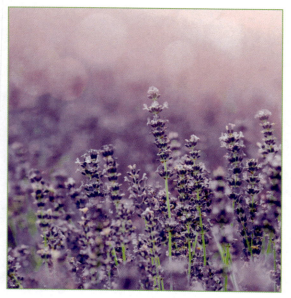

Lavender

Sleep issues, stress, anxiety, teeth grinding, sunburns, burns, scars, allergies and hay fever, colic and upset baby, cuts, wounds, blisters, bug bites, hives, nosebleeds, pink eye, high blood pressure, migraines and headaches, emotional balance

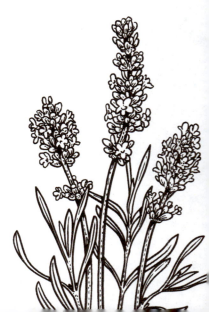

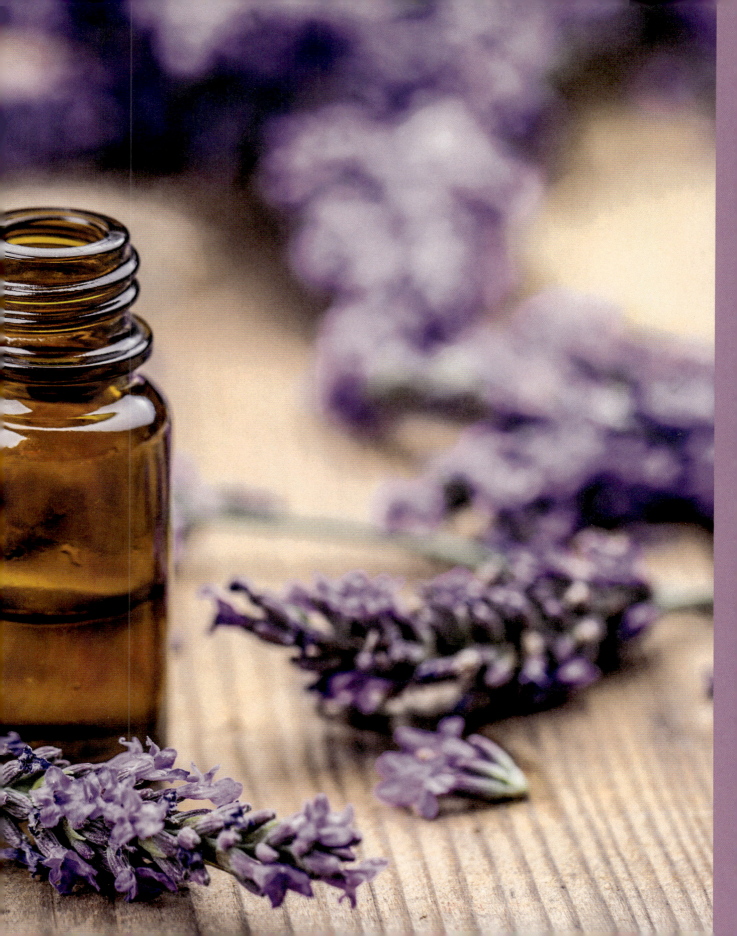

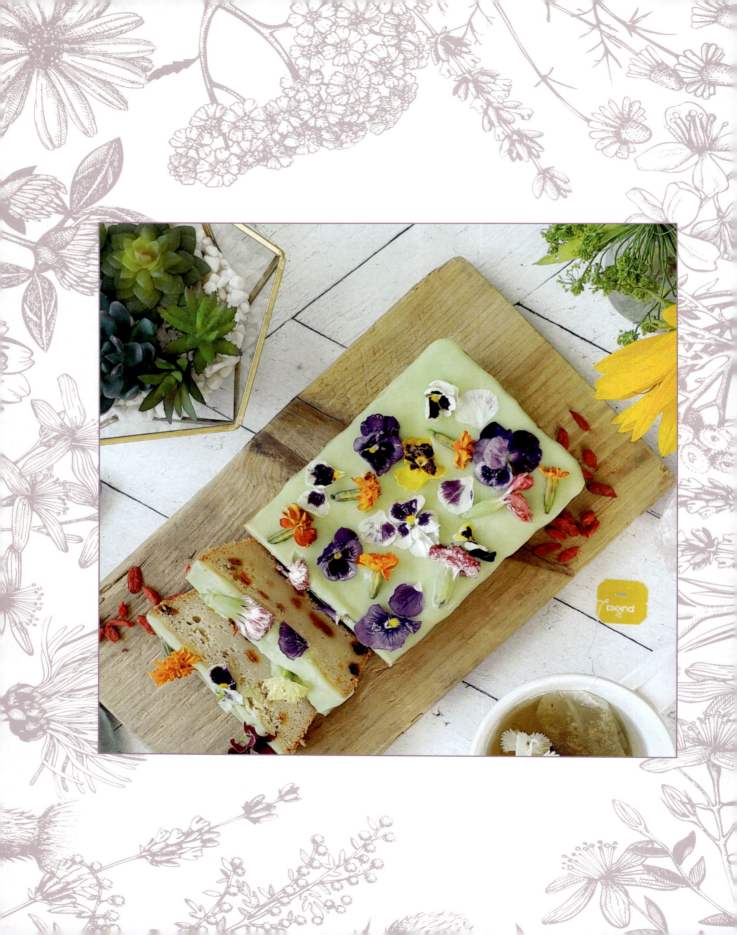

AROMA: *GREEN + FLORAL* | **FLAVORS:** *SWEET + EARTHY*
PAIRS WITH: *CITRUS* | **MAIN USES:** *BEAUTIFY*

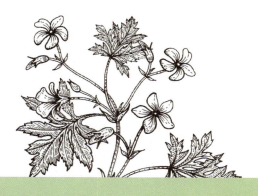

Geranium

FLOWER POWER POUND CAKE

1/4 cup melted coconut oil
200 mL almond milk
3 T apple cider vinegar
1/2 cup maple syrup
1 t vanilla

1 1/4 cup almond flour
1 1/4 cup GF flour
pinch salt
1 T baking powder
1/2 t baking soda

2 drops Geranium essential oil
1 drop Lavender essential oil

1/4 cup melted coconut butter
2 T agave
1/4 t vanilla

1. Combine the liquids in a medium bowl, one that is also large enough to incorporate the dry ingredients.
2. Combine the dry ingredients in a separate bowl and sift them into the bowl with the wet ingredients. Mix gently until just combined.
3. Add the essential oils just before baking at 325°F for 50-60 minutes.
4. Make a glaze by melting 1/4 cup coconut butter. Add 1-2 T agave, 1/4 t vanilla, and one drop of lavender essential oil, thinning with hot water until thin enough to spread. Optional to add natural food color before glazing.
5. Once baked, cool the loaf in the pan for 5 minutes before removing to cool completely.
6. Spread the glaze over the top and let it drip down the sides. Top with edible flowers and goji berries. Refrigerate to set the glaze before slicing and serving.

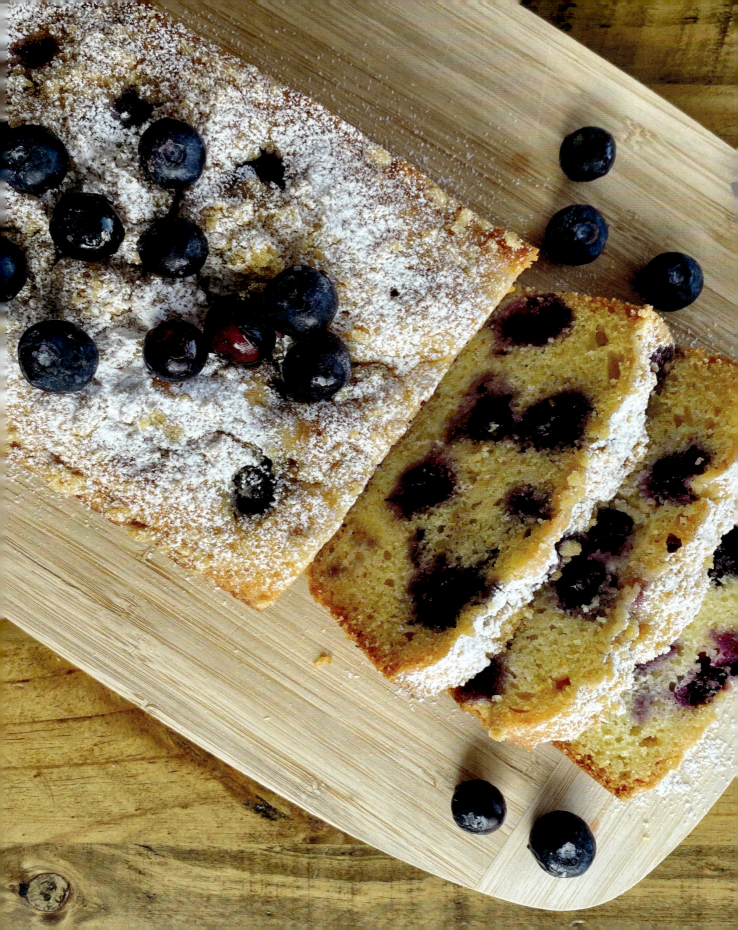

AROMA: *LIGHT and FLORAL* | **FLAVORS:** *PUNGENT and FLORAL*
PAIRS WITH: *VANILLA and LEMON* | **MAIN USES:** *RELAXING*

Lavender

BLUEBERRY LAVENDER BREAD

1/4 cup melted coconut oil
200 mL almond milk
3 T apple cider vinegar
1/2 cup maple syrup
1 t vanilla

1 1/4 cup almond flour
1 1/4 cup GF flour
Pinch salt
1 T baking powder
1/2 t baking soda

2 drops Lavender essential oil
1 cup frozen blueberries

1/4 cup melted coconut butter
2 T agave
1/2 t vanilla
1 drop Lavender essential oil

1. Combine the liquids in a medium bowl, one that is also large enough to incorporate the dry ingredients.
2. Combine the dry ingredients in a separate bowl and sift them into the bowl with the wet ingredients. Mix gently until just combined.
3. Add the lavender essential oil just before baking at 325°F for 50-60 minutes.
4. Make a glaze by melting 1/4 cup coconut butter. Add 1-2 T agave, vanilla, and one drop of lavender essential oil, thinning with hot water until thin enough to spread. Optional to add natural food color before glazing.
5. Once baked, cool the loaf in the pan for 5 minutes before removing to cool completely.
6. Spread the glaze over the top and let it drip down the sides. Top with sliced almonds. Refrigerate to set the glaze before slicing and serving.

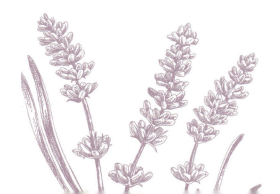

LAVENDER CHOCOLATE TRUFFLES

1 can coconut milk, refrigerated overnight—use top cream only
1 bag dairy free chocolate chips
1 drop Lavender essential oil

1. Melt coconut cream and chocolate chips until smooth. Stir in essential oil and refrigerate until firm but still soft enough to scoop into truffles.
2. Roll in cacao powder, coconut flakes, chopped nuts, or a mixture! Store in refrigerator.

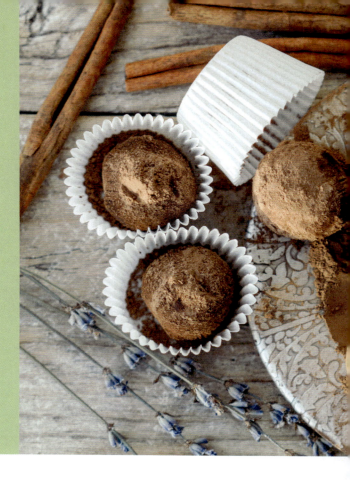

VANILLA LAVENDER MOON MILK

1 cup oat milk, warmed
1 T almond butter
1 T maple syrup or local honey
Drop of vanilla extract or use a small piece of vanilla bean
Dash of nutmeg
Pinch of salt

Blend in a high-powered blender until smooth and frothy. Stir in Lavender essential oil 1 toothpick at a time until desired potency is reached.

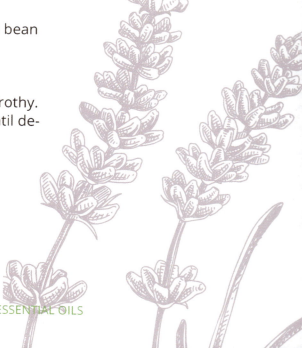

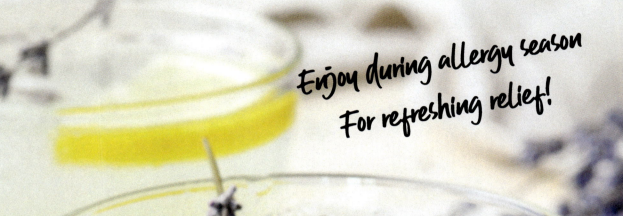

Enjoy during allergy season for refreshing relief!

LAVENDER LEMONADE

1 T hot water
1 t local honey
2 T lemon juice
8 oz cold water, still or sparkling

Melt the honey in hot water before adding lemon juice and water. Stir in Lavender oil 1 toothpick at a time until desired potency is reached.

Acknowledgments

Katarina, thank you for your patience, support, and attention to detail in taking the photos for this book. Your ability to capture the beauty of these recipes with such ease was a much-needed collaboration that I didn't know I needed. Photoshoot days were one of my favorite aspects of this project, and I am so truly grateful to have had you so involved.

Kattrina, thank you for loaning the beautiful dishware for our photoshoots! Your generosity is so very appreciated.

Nancy, Franzi, and Tricia, thank you for helping me realize my avenue to share the power of essential oils! You are all such an inspiration in your own unique way. I am so grateful for your friendship, advice, encouragement, support, and so much more.

Mom and Dad, thank you for guiding my culinary curiosity. All of those classes, camps, programs and cookbooks have been the gluten-free vegan breadcrumbs that helped me discover this purpose. For allowing me to determine the pace with which I pursue this lifelong passion, and for stoking the fire when I need it, I am so very grateful. Your support of this lifestyle means the world.

Kyle, thank you for helping me eat all of the recipes, even the ones that didn't come out as intended. For being as excited as I was when a recipe worked, and dancing with me in delicious victory. Your patience, kindness, and willingness to listen as I navigated through the ups and downs of this creative process is one of the major reasons that this book even exists. I am eternally grateful.

Astara Jane Ashley and Flower of Life Press, a thousand thank you's for holding space for me to explore my inner world as reflected by my outer world and life circumstances. Your wisdom, patience, guidance, and compassion are such incredible natural assets which made the creative process a truly divine journey. I am forever grateful for all of the ways that you have inspired me to show up and serve by stepping back into authenticity and alignment. Thank you for helping me to bring this book into the world, for the endless hours spent making all of the edits, and for being my publishing expert in manifesting this book.

Additional books by Lauren D'Agostino

Available at **www.laurendagostino.com/shop**

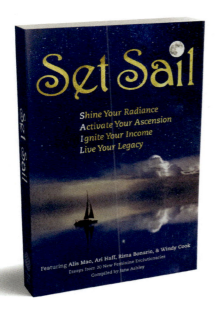

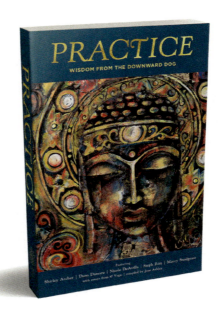

Set Sail: Shine Your Radiance, Activate Your Ascension, Ignite Your Income, Live Your Legacy

Practice: Wisdom from the Downward Dog

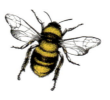

Additional books by Flower of Life Press

The New Feminine Evolutionary: Embody Presence—Become the Change

Pioneering the Path to Prosperity: Discover the Power of True Wealth
and Abundance

Sacred Body Wisdom: Igniting the Flame of Our Divine Humanity

Emerge: 7 Steps to Transformation (No matter what life throws at you!)

Sisterhood of the Mindful Goddess: How to Remove Obstacles, Activate Your Gifts,
and Become Your Own Superhero

Path of the Priestess: Discover Your Divine Purpose

Sacred Call of the Ancient Priestess: Birthing a New Feminine Archetype

Rise Above: Free Your Mind One Brushstroke at a Time

Menopause Mavens: Master the Mystery of Menopause

The Power of Essential Oils: Create Positive Transformation in
Your Well-Being, Business, and Life

Self-Made Wellionaire: Get Off Your Ass(et), Reclaim Your Health,
and Feel Like a Million Bucks

Oms From the Mat: Breathe, Move, and Awaken to the Power of Yoga

Oms From the Heart: Open Your Heart to the Power of Yoga

The Four Tenets of Love: Open, Activate, and Inspire Your Life's Path

The Fire-Driven Life: Ignite the Fire of Self-Worth, Health, and Happiness with a
Plant-Based Diet

Becoming Enough: A Heroine's Journey to the Already Perfect Self

The Unfucked Code: Transform Your Relationships from Fighting to Uniting

The Caregiving Journey: Information. Guidance. Inspiration.

Visit us **at www.FlowerofLifepress.com**

Made in the USA
Middletown, DE
11 May 2021